Joshua s world

Joshua's World

Hermione Woodley

ISBN-13: 978-1482700374
ISBN-10: 1482700379

DEDICATION

To my children who have taught me so much

CONTENTS

ACKNOWLEDGMENTS

So many people have played a part in caring for Joshua. Each individual has brought something unique. Thank you all so much for your love, support and time. I would also like to thank my husband, who has walked this path with me. Finally, I want to mention my mother whose prayers for Joshua have been invaluable.

1 PLEASE NOT THIS WAY!

The days trickle by
Some more eventful than others
I allow myself to settle in the routine called 'our life'.

Life is good, life is calm
Surely we are safe in our tomorrows
The future that is all planned out in my mind

But who is this unexpected intruder
That has suddenly appeared in our midst?

There is a shadow that it seems to cast over us
I am faced with a feeling of dread.

I do not know where it has come from
Or even how long it will stay

All I know is that it was not invited
All I can do now is hope and pray

I am now straining to see all of our tomorrows
Everything now seems hazy and vague

So what is the required response from us?
Is it simply come what may?

  I wonder, does the term 'special needs' mean
anything to you? Is there a total blank when you hear

the phrase, or does an image or perhaps a memory invade your mind? The term itself can mean something different to each individual and each family affected. Each single experience of 'special needs' is of course unlike any other, with the nature of those needs varying from person to person. So much encompassed in such a short phrase; so many interpretations. A world of such diversity! No longer ordinary but 'special'. If your family is affected, by someone who falls into this category, then your experience will be unique; no other family will be going through exactly what your own is going through. There are always those out there who are going through similar experiences. They may have stories like your own to tell and it is perhaps these people we can empathize with the most. Often, it is therapeutic to share with and encourage each other because we are all on our own journey and at times it can be lonely. Lives might be changed forever but for some it may be just for a season. We can never truly understand how individuals or families are really affected. We may notice the outward changes but we never know the full extent. We see only what is visible on the outside. Your perspective is dependent on your vantage point. Are you in the thick of it? Are you someone caring for a special needs person? Perhaps you are growing up with a special needs sibling? Maybe you are the friend of a family who is going through it right now and you are at a loss as to how you can help. You might be a grandparent feeling for both your own child and your grandchild. Life changes and relationships are perhaps strained.

As for us, our experience brings to the surface a

whole host of feelings and memories. Our journey has taken me down pathways that I never even knew existed. The experience can make me want to cry and laugh at the same time. Having a child with special needs has changed my perspective on life and broadened my outlook. It has also catapulted me into deep despair at times and forced me to grow as a person. Circumstances have made me stop, reassess the world around me through different eyes and decide afresh what I now consider to be important. I see people in different ways now. Perhaps this is because I am more aware of the needs of those around me. I have been stopped in my tracks and forced to deviate from the pathway that I thought I was meant to be on. I have been made to stand still and take a long look at some of those very special people who fall into this unique category of individuals. Mind you, it is hardly a single group because those who are set apart by their special needs are as diverse as the range of colours that exist. No two shades are quite the same with special needs, as even those who have the same diagnosis will not be identical. Yes, there is overlap but their needs are theirs alone because they are indeed unique.

There have always been people with special needs and I know I have noticed them and even felt for them. I wonder if I was really seeing them. I remember as a child feeling very emotional whenever I passed someone collecting for the disadvantaged or the sick. I would always ask my mother for money to put into the collection tin. Long after they were out of sight they would still be on my mind. Eventually the picture in my mind would fade as the distance between us grew. Special needs had only ever crossed my path briefly. A very good friend of mine had a severely handicapped sister. Looking back I remember the family as being among the kindest and most tender-hearted people I have ever met. Was their perspective on life different to mine? It was not the same for my husband Mark. 'Special needs' had not just brushed past him but was a part of his everyday life, while growing up. His younger brother has Down's syndrome.

I can remember a time when there was really nothing out of the ordinary about our life. We were the parents of three boys and they all appeared to be developing normally. However, that changed when my third son Joshua reached the age of about one and a half years old. Life was, as to be expected, a little hectic with three young children but Mark and I enjoyed being parents, and all that parenthood brought with it! Life was forever changing and we did our best to deal with the challenges that came our way. Joshua, like his brothers, was a lovely looking little boy. At first he didn't appear to look anything like his siblings at all. They have deep brown eyes and Joshua was the first of our children to be born with blue eyes. Also, unlike his brothers, he had straight fair hair in contrast to the black curly hair of his siblings. However, if you took the time to look closely you could definitely see the resemblance. So here was our Joshua, who it has to be said was a bit of a textbook baby really, a good-natured, placid and healthy boy. Joshua ate well, slept well and was a very responsive, affectionate baby who appeared to enjoy having people around him. When he was born it was as though he had always been with us and he seemed to adjust to our busy lifestyle with ease. Soon he started babbling and was attempting to say his first words. The children's T.V. character 'Bob the Builder' was a huge hit with him. Joshua would entertain us by trying to 'sing' the theme song, from quite an early age. I remember us all being so proud of him and we would always request an encore! He, like most babies, enjoyed it when his brothers played peek-a-boo with him or tickled him. At that time he certainly came across as a baby who was clearly interacting with and exploring the world around him, right up until the age of about one and a half, that is! We had no idea of what was lurking around the corner which was probably just as well. It wasn't until we were expecting our fourth child that we began to suspect that there might be a problem. Physically Joshua's development was like that of any other toddler but in some areas he seemed to have stopped moving forward. It wasn't blatantly obvious though because he was such an easy child to manage. It was more the little things that could very easily be missed. For example, he didn't wave goodbye or even say goodbye unless prompted to. People would generally put this down to shyness. However, more alarmingly, he soon stopped babbling altogether. He no longer attempted to sing 'Bob the builder' and he seemed to retreat into a place deep within himself. Looking back, it definitely wasn't any one thing in particular but it was just a vague notion that only a parent would spot initially. We both tried to dismiss the fears but they refused to lie and instead darted about at the back of our minds. But as is often said, 'life goes on,' and the days seemed to fly by dragging all of our concerns along with them. Soon we were all immersed in the preparation for baby number four and all the excitement surrounding the event. Joshua was just two years old when our daughter was born. Although he was not really aware of what was happening, his brothers were both caught up in the anticipation of our new arrival. Megan caused much excitement when she was born and she, like Joshua, has gorgeous blue eyes. Joshua was now no longer the baby of the family but there was certainly no jealousy, on his part, mainly because he didn't seem to register her existence. The fact that we had become a family of six seemed to bypass him totally. His lack of reaction was in direct contrast to that of his brothers who could barely contain their excitement at having another baby in the house; to crown it all it was a girl! They gave her such a wonderful welcome home when we brought her back from the hospital. Mark and I joined them in their elation and we really felt as though our family was now complete. The novelty of having lots of girly paraphernalia dotted around the house was quite something to behold. It was a welcomed distraction from our concerns for Joshua, which festered away at the back of our minds. I chatted to our health visitor about my misgivings. Our suspicions were mostly caused by the fact that Joshua was still not trying to communicate, verbally or otherwise. Every so often he would be a bit more responsive but it never seemed to last very long. The health visitor didn't appear to be overly worried because he was still very young. She was of the opinion that, being our third child, his brothers probably did a lot of the talking for him. Also, during the visit, not only had Joshua noticed the health visitor but he had approached her, made eye contact and touched her arm! However, since I had raised the issue of his slower development, especially when compared to his brothers, she arranged to see Joshua again in a few months' time, to check his progress. She was very kind and in the meantime she did her best to alleviate our fears. People kept saying that he was fine but, although we so wanted to believe it, we were just not convinced. We tried to be positive and to push through all of those niggling doubts but, try as we might, they just would not rest. Questions and thoughts kept surfacing... Why was he no longer responding to his name? Why was there only fleeting eye contact? Why was he so quiet? And so the questions bounced back and forth. Time did not seem to be a healer, for him or for us. With each passing day Joshua appeared to be retreating even more into his own quiet world. He didn't seem to be particularly bothered if he was in a room on his own or if he was in a room packed with children. It was as though he was really somewhere else anyway and so the presence of other children didn't seem to register with him at all. He was happy enough to play alongside other children but communicate with them he would not! However, on a positive note, he was content when left in the crèche at church or at a friend's house if the need arose. He was one of those children who you could leave knowing that he wouldn't be any trouble. As long as there were toys to play with he was fine. He never grabbed toys from other children and oddly enough he didn't make a fuss when they were taken out of his hands either, which was most unusual for a toddler. Young children normally show their displeasure in some way but Joshua never did. I used to hope that he would learn to be a bit more assertive. I certainly didn't want him to go around hitting other children or anything like that. It was just that he never tried to retrieve anything taken from him and his face did not even indicate that he was upset. I was becoming more and more concerned.

Again we spoke to our health visitor who listened. It was suggested that maybe Joshua simply couldn't hear properly, as he just wasn't responding to the spoken word. Hearing tests were then arranged. I was relieved to see that some action was being taken. The tests were difficult to carry out because it was hard to get Joshua to stay on task. It was usually when we were in a situation outside the home, where Joshua was required to follow instructions, that it became painfully obvious just how delayed he was. This was definitely one of those occasions. Nevertheless they persevered and as it turned out, the tests showed that Joshua did in fact have significant glue ear. At last we thought we had some sort of reason or even an answer! More importantly we now had an explanation that we could give to people. Following his initial hearing test, he was referred to the Ear, Nose & Throat (ENT) clinic at the hospital where they would carry out more in-depth hearing tests. In the meantime all we could do was to wait for his appointments. The health visitor had also referred him to the speech and language services and sometime later Joshua received an appointment. Now I felt that we had something other than the problem to focus on. Joshua needed all the help he could get and we were keen to be as actively involved as we could be. The speech therapist spent some time getting to know Joshua and tried to interact with him through play. Although Joshua didn't appear the least bit concerned with his peers, he loved toys and she had an abundance of them in her room! Joshua was soon totally absorbed in seeking out the tractors, trailers, trains and cars (essentially anything with wheels!). She confirmed that he was indeed much delayed in his speech for his age, but on a positive note said that the sounds that he was making were all the right ones. This was good news and it gave us hope that Joshua's communication skills would improve with time. At that point one of my greatest fears was that Joshua would never talk and so I was relieved when she said that he would probably be verbal in time. The appointment with the speech therapist brought a certain amount of relief but still my concerns for Joshua's future were not allayed. Although fear of the unknown seemed to be holding us hostage, we were determined to hold on tightly to anything positive. In the meantime the days went by and Joshua appeared contented enough. It was true that he did not interact with his peers but he continued to be very loving towards Mark and myself. Like any child he would play with his toys and like most children he had his favourites. Naturally he seemed very quiet because he wasn't vocal and at times appeared completely withdrawn from the rest of the family. However, at the same time, we felt a certain amount of reassurance because he was so affectionate and he seemed most content when he was being held. This was something that I took great comfort in. You see even then the word 'autism' was at the back of my mind. Strange really because I didn't have a clue what autism really meant; neither had I met anyone with autism. I don't know why the word was invading my thinking, but it was. 'Surely the fact that Joshua is so loving and tactile means it can't possibly be autism?' Mark and I would ask ourselves. Our perception of autism was based on the snippets of information that we had got mainly from television. Autistic characters were not normally depicted as being overly demonstrative. Mark and I had dared to mention our fears to a few people who seemed to be of the same opinion. 'No he is fine,' they would say. 'He is just a bit delayed that is all. Once the glue ear is sorted out he will be a different child.' We were certainly not about to argue with that! How totally wrong we were. It is so true what they say, 'Ignorance is bliss!'

The weeks trickled by and there were days when Joshua's problems seemed hardly noticeable. As an onlooker you probably wouldn't have thought anything was wrong at all but then, out of the blue, there would be a situation which would really distress him in a way that just wasn't normal. Of course we attributed this to the glue ear because he would sometimes get very upset when confronted with lots of noise. On one occasion, while on holiday in Scotland, we thought it would be fun to visit a sea life centre there. As soon as we arrived Joshua seemed uncomfortable but when we were all inside, for reasons only known to him, he became absolutely hysterical. It was so upsetting to see him like that because we could not understand the cause of his distress. We felt that other than removing him from the situation, for a while, there was very little we could do. When you have other children it is not always possible, or fair on them, to just up and leave. We would usually try to calm Joshua down by distracting him, or by whatever other means we thought best. If that failed we would remove him, for a short while, and then gradually reintroduce him. It usually worked and eventually, after reassuring him, he would settle down and we could continue with what we were doing. This time however Joshua was having none of it. (I seem to recall Joshua reacting in a similar manner on a trip to the circus. It was also fairly dark in there and nothing would persuade him to stay in the big top. He was simply terrified.) Any parent will know that it is always a challenge when you are confronted with a baby in distress, who is obviously unable to communicate their needs to you other than by crying. So it was with Joshua at times. There were occasions during this period when Joshua would just sob uncontrollably, but he did not have the language to communicate to us what was bothering him. He was about two and a half years old at this time. It was so hard to see him upset and yet be unable to make things better for him. As a parent it goes against all of your natural instincts. Joshua had been a child who you could take pretty much anywhere, but he was gradually changing into someone who found certain situations, noises and environments intolerable. We still had no idea why. It was difficult to predict exactly what would trigger a reaction from Joshua so it wasn't simply a case of avoiding certain places. If he were at a crowded soft play area for instance he would have loved it. He would quite happily dive into the ball pit or go down the huge slide. He didn't even mind going down the enclosed slide. It made no sense to us at all. These 'instances' however were still quite rare so we just dealt with them as best as we could.

Joshua's birthday seemed to be rapidly approaching. He would be three in August. At the back of our minds was the fact that he was due to start nursery in September, but he did not seem at all ready. He was normally with me when his brother was dropped off. Occasionally Joshua and his sister would attend a party, bazaar or some other event there, so it was not unfamiliar territory. We had all been to the Christmas party there and had a great time. Naturally when the Easter party came around, I thought it would be a fun activity to share with Joshua and Megan. Nothing could have prepared me for Joshua's reaction. There was of course an Easter bonnet parade and all sorts of other things going on; it should have been lovely. As a surprise for the children, the T.V. characters the 'Tweenies' were to put in an appearance (in reality some committee members dressed up in 'Tweenies' costumes). Under normal circumstances Joshua loved the 'Tweenies' so his reaction could not have been predicted. He became very distressed. I held him close and whispered into his ear, 'Joshua darling it's ok I'm here.' However, soon he was completely hysterical. He was making so much noise that I had no choice but to take him out of the room and eventually back to the car. The normal method of removing him, followed by a gradual reintroduction to the scene, did not work on this occasion. I really didn't feel it was right to disrupt the party with the noise that Joshua was making. He was simply inconsolable. I couldn't explain why he had reacted like that, but I put it down to the larger than life costumes that he was confronted with. Not a very good introduction to nursery, I thought to myself! I tried not to worry but I felt increasingly uneasy, as well as a bit embarrassed that it was my child who was disrupting the proceedings. Common sense told me that what was troubling Joshua was more than just glue ear. Joshua's unusual behaviour could certainly not be attributed to glue ear alone. Deep down I think I had known this all along, but I was loath to admit it to myself. To admit it meant that I would have to confront it and ultimately deal with it; I just was not ready for that. So called 'normal' life was becoming hard work and activities that we had once taken for granted were now battles to be overcome. Swimming, for example, became difficult for us to enjoy as a family. Joshua would start to cry as soon as we were in the car park. He would still be screaming by the time we had managed to change and get into the pool. He was simply petrified and once in the water would cling to myself or his dad. Mark and I would take turns to calm him in the water, while the other concentrated on the remaining children. After several minutes in the water it was as though he would realise that it was ok and that he was safe. Slowly he would settle down, start to relax and then he would actually enjoy his time in the pool. Taking young children swimming always involves effort but with Joshua in the equation it was even harder work. So what were we to do? We didn't want to stop going swimming as a family and felt that it was important that we encouraged him to push through his fear. Again it wasn't obvious what caused him to react like this. Was it his glue ear or perhaps a sensory issue? We didn't know, but when he had calmed down he actually had a great time. Admittedly it would have been easier to avoid swimming altogether. In doing so we would have reduced all of our stress levels, but we knew that despite his initial reaction he loved water. For his own safety he needed to learn to swim.

Delaying the inevitable was not going to help. Although Joshua was still on the whole a fairly placid child, he was definitely becoming more difficult to manage in certain situations. We noticed that for instance it became harder to keep him quiet when you needed to and it was impossible to keep him confined to one activity, or one area, for any length of time. If he was at a soft play area or outside he was fine because he loved to climb, jump and bounce. However if he needed to sit and play a game with other children, e.g. pass the parcel, he found it a challenge. There was one particular party I remember Joshua and I having to leave early. He just couldn't understand any of the party games and so was not remotely interested in joining in. In the next room he could see the party food all spread out on a table. However, for reasons that he couldn't fathom, he was unable to eat any of it. To make matters worse he had noticed a little park area outside and that was where he really wanted to be. All of the other children were having fun as their parents looked on proudly. I, on the other hand, was repeating a series of phases to Joshua such as, 'sit down!' or, 'No Joshua, don't do that!' He was into absolutely anything and everything and he didn't seem to comprehend the concept of NO, in any shape or form! You could tell Joshua not to touch something and moments later he would be back there again, and again, AND AGAIN! I was silently willing Joshua to comply and in doing so to fit in, but he wasn't going to and that was that. I could feel the embarrassment taking root as the other mothers stared. Eventually I apologised and took him home. It wasn't fair to make him stay when he was clearly struggling and definitely not enjoying himself.

Looking back, I remember running around after Joshua far more than I ever had to for his siblings. This was not only because of the usual things that toddlers would get up to but because Joshua had the knack of touching, destroying, eating and generally picking up anything that he wasn't supposed to. He would feast on play doh whenever he got the opportunity and he was very skilled at sneaking a piece into his mouth, before you even realised that he had done it. He could eat several little portions with you sitting at the table next to him. He was swift, determined and had impeccable timing. Joshua would wait for you to look away for just a nanosecond (or so it seemed) and before you could do anything a little piece of play doh was making its way down into his tummy. You would think that it would have made him sick but no, he truly had (and still has for that matter) a cast iron stomach. He is the only child I know who can sneak pieces of raw bacon and it has no noticeable effect on him! Apparently paint was also a rather tasty dish. You would be lulled into a false sense of security, by the fact that he was using a paintbrush and paper appropriately, but as soon as he could he would stick the paint brush into his mouth. Yuk! Other regular snacks included dirt, stones, uncooked rice or pasta and sand, to mention but a few. At first I thought that it was just a phase that he was going through, because most children go through a stage of putting things in their mouths. For Joshua though, he seemed to be stuck at that point and it lasted for a long time. I dread to think how much play doh Joshua has eaten over the years!

All of my children have a real love of the outdoors and Joshua is no exception. It is great when Joshua can play outside, because it is good for him to use up some of that energy of which he seems to have an abundant supply! He loves to run, climb trees, trampoline and go on the swings or slide. However, there was a downside to letting Joshua play in the garden when he was going through his phase of shoving everything into his mouth. There were countless times, when Joshua was playing outside, that I would notice him munching on a mouthful of dirt. He would then have to be taken inside and cleaned up. On one occasion a friend had dropped in and we were chatting. This was before Megan was born; in fact I was pregnant with her at the time. It was a beautiful sunny day and we were watching Joshua playing. He seemed to be having a great time and he didn't appear to be doing anything that he wasn't supposed to be doing. Lulled into a false sense of security I sat down for a moment and had some of my tea. Taking that as his cue Joshua came in from the garden, through the patio doors. I frowned at him because I noticed that his hands were covered in what I thought was dirt. But 'Hey this is progress,' I thought to myself, 'At least it hasn't got as far as his mouth this time. Maybe he is starting to realise that dirt isn't such a good thing to eat after all.' The strange thing was that he was holding his hands out to me, as though he definitely didn't want to put what looked like dirt in his mouth. When he got closer I soon realised why. It wasn't dirt at all it was cat's poo! He had clearly drawn the line at that for which I have to say I was relieved. It was bad enough that he had got it all over his hands and had to be thoroughly cleaned but at least he hadn't eaten it. Cat's poo is not something that you relish cleaning up anyway, especially when you are pregnant! However, that was the first and last time that Joshua ever touched the stuff. Phew!

Following the disastrous Easter party, spring seemed to race by. It wasn't until the beginning of the summer holidays that we received a date for Joshua's hospital appointment, at the ENT clinic. The appointments were scheduled for October which meant more waiting. This was not soon enough, as far as we were concerned, because Joshua was due to start nursery in September and he still wasn't talking. To complicate the situation further he was still in nappies and showed absolutely no signs of wanting to use the toilet. We contacted the hospital to see if there was any chance that he could be seen sooner. After several phone calls we realised that there was no flexibility there. So there was no choice but to wait. As far as nursery was concerned there was nothing we could do until the beginning of term. We planned to take him in then and explain that, due to his problems, it would not be possible for him to start. Since Joshua would not be seen before term started we now had nothing definite to tell them. The doctors had talked about Joshua having grommets fitted when the glue ear was initially detected. However, he was considered too young at that point. It was decided that the situation would be reviewed when he was next seen. The month of September crept up on us and before I knew it the children were back to school. It was also the day that Joshua was due to start nursery. As I got Joshua ready I wished that we had talked to the nursery beforehand. I suppose, deep down, we had both hoped that Joshua's problems would have been on their way to being resolved by then. I had already decided in my head that he definitely would not be starting that day and it all seemed a bit pointless taking him along really. However, it wasn't something I wanted to discuss with the nursery staff over the telephone. 'Besides,' I told myself, 'Joshua was probably one of those children who would benefit from starting nursery later. Surely he would catch up eventually, wouldn't he?' Mark and I arrived at the nursery and explained to the lady in charge. We told her about the glue ear, his lack of speech and the fact that he wasn't toilet trained. Neither Mark nor I could have anticipated her response. She suggested that we try leaving Joshua for the morning to see how he got on. We were both thrown! We certainly hadn't come expecting to leave him there. We were slightly apprehensive because he wasn't exactly happy to be there, but also because we wondered how he would make his needs known to them. As his parents we could normally work out what he needed, because we were used to his ways, but even we didn't always get it right. We knew what he was likely to get up to and what he would try to touch. How on earth would they cope with him? We didn't want to throw him or them in at the deep end, but on the other hand it wasn't going to do Joshua any good at all if we were overly protective. So we agreed to let him stay for the morning, to see how he liked it, and off we went leaving our very distressed little boy. It felt odd; he had only ever been left with someone who we knew well. Although I had been through the first day at nursery scenario with his brothers this felt very different. They didn't have the problems that he had. They had understanding and they could voice their concerns. They could tell me about their day. Joshua on the other hand couldn't. In many ways he was like a baby, in that you still had to do so much for him, and the understanding was just not there.

Two and a half hours later we were waiting nervously with the other parents to collect him. Well he was still in once piece and what was more they were too! They had managed to calm him down and he had apparently enjoyed his morning, we were told. They said that he didn't take a lot of notice of the other children but he wasn't particularly bothered by their presence either. They also noted that he tended to flit from one activity to another which sounded exactly like Joshua. The lady in charge even said that it really didn't matter that he was still in nappies. They were happy for him to attend and they suggested that we talked again, after he had been to the hospital for his appointments. We were absolutely staggered by their response. When they realised that he was going to need constant supervision, they took it upon themselves to have an extra member of staff on hand just to 'Josh watch' as they called it. Amazing! To begin with they did not even receive any extra funding for the one to one support that Joshua received. Although we did offer to cover this they wouldn't hear of it! Their reaction was a true reflection of the caring environment that they provided for the children. The atmosphere in the nursery was warm and they seemed to have a genuine concern for Joshua. We were more than happy to leave him in their capable hands and we really received this as God's provision for our son.

After a short while Joshua became more accustomed to his routine at nursery and he loved going there. The members of staff were daily recipients of his cuddles and they really did seem to go beyond the call of duty. All that remained was for us to wait for Joshua's hospital appointments. So a new routine started to take shape in our household. Joshua would be dropped off at nursery two mornings a week. For the first time since my daughter was born I had regular slots where it was just the two of us and these occasions were precious. I also found that I was able to relax in a way that I just couldn't when Joshua was around. By now of course, we were well aware of Joshua's problems and when I collected him from nursery his difficulties seemed to be highlighted all the more. I couldn't help but feel self-conscious. Just seeing your 'special' child, with all their struggles, alongside normally functioning children tends to accentuate their unusual behaviour. At nursery Joshua was always the one who was doing his own thing. He would be the one who couldn't sit for the story, or the child I could hear before I could see him through the doors.

2 DIAGNOSIS

Autism was still at the back of my mind and although I had no clear idea what it actually was I did know that it was serious. I began to look up 'autism' on the internet just to find out exactly what the term meant. I suppose I was hoping that, once I had looked it up, I would find that Joshua's problems were nothing like those with which autism was associated. Mentally I could then cross autism off the invisible list in my head. Well that may have been what I was looking for, but it certainly wasn't what I got. According to my research, people with autism have three main areas of difficulty in common. These are sometimes known as the 'triad of impairments'. What did this all mean exactly? It didn't make a huge amount of sense to me and so I kept reading. Apparently the core problem in autism is social and, as a result, those people affected find it extremely hard to understand the world around them. The first of these three impairments is with social communication. It would appear that autistic individuals do not understand fully the purpose or meaning of language, and struggle with both verbal and non-verbal communication. Some may have no speech at all or their language may be very limited. Others may have excellent language skills, but still not really understand the mechanics of a conversation. They may fail to see that it is two way and just talk at you about something that interests them. Sometimes they may simply repeat what has been said to them.

This is known as 'echolalia'. Certain phrases may be taken literally and body language is easily missed. The second difficulty is with social interaction. Individuals with autism generally find that socialising does not come naturally. They miss the unwritten social codes of behaviour and they literally have to be learnt. It is difficult for them to understand other people's emotions and feelings. They can also have trouble expressing their own and so find it difficult to 'fit in'. These challenges can make it hard for them to strike up a friendship. The third difficulty is to do with social imagination. This ability allows us to comprehend and to predict other people's behaviour, grasp abstract ideas and to picture unfamiliar situations. Autistic individuals find it hard to comprehend and decode other people's thoughts, emotions and behaviour. They find it tricky to anticipate what might happen next. This is probably why people with autism have a limited concept of danger. They are unable to look ahead and predict what could happen if they were to just wander off, or run into a busy road. It can also be hard for an autistic child to engage in imaginative play. They may prefer to re-enact the same scene over and over. Impaired social imagination can make it difficult to cope with change or unfamiliar situations. (Problems with social imagination, however, do not mean a lack of imagination.)

Autism is said to be part of the autistic spectrum. As the word 'spectrum' indicates, the exact degree to which each person is affected will vary from one to another. All of those on the spectrum will have the problems which are described as the 'triad of impairments'. However each individual will be affected in different ways and to different degrees. It seemed to me that autistic individuals find the world of people hard to fathom. To an onlooker it might appear that they lack the so called 'common-sense' that we take for granted. Autistic children can sometimes be perceived as naughty because they are often misunderstood. There is so much yet to be discovered about the world of autism. It affects a group of people who do not necessarily look any different from you and me. However, their behaviours often set them apart. For instance, autistic individuals can sometimes respond in unusual ways to sensory stimuli.

I took a sharp intake of breath as I read on. Autism was described as a developmental disability that was present from birth, but not always immediately apparent. It was a life-long disability for which there was no cure. No wait, hold on a minute, surely no cure must mean no hope! End of the road. What do you do with that? How do you live with no hope? I needed to stop reading because my head was dizzy from the invasion of unwanted facts. Was this really Joshua's problem? I didn't know and, to be honest, at that moment it was better not to know. The reality was that I could not erase all of those details from my mind despite my efforts. This unwelcome information was like some sort of leach which had now attached itself to my thinking. Feelings of dread started to come over me and I was afraid. At whose door could I lay down all my fears? At that time, to voice my suspicions to anyone other than Mark would have been like breathing life into something, which was at that stage merely a possibility, somewhere in my thinking. To speak it out would almost be like giving it form and substance. Although I couldn't be completely open with anyone else, I knew I could be open with God. Somehow I could accept that He understood completely what I was feeling. He knew that there were times when I felt totally alone in it all and so very scared of the unknown. He knew how difficult it was for us to wait. I couldn't even contemplate how I would begin to accept a diagnosis of autism, so I tried not to dwell on it. There was nothing that I could do but pray. My prayers at that time were desperate and anxious ones and Joshua's needs were all I could see. They were just like a huge black cloud that seemed to be blotting out the sun in our lives. It was as though our days were being swallowed up by this oppressive gloom. God didn't remove the source of the pain. The problem didn't just disappear. Instead I found that, just when I felt I couldn't take it anymore, my whole being would be soothed by a peace that could only have come from God. He would remind me gently that, although I often felt alone in it all, He was right there with us and that was where He was going to stay. I clung to His faithfulness; I had to. For us being members of a church family made so much difference. We knew that we were not going through this on our own, regardless of how we felt. Many, many prayers went up for Joshua and for us as a family. At that time, I held on to the vague hope that when Joshua went for his appointments they would give us a totally different diagnosis. In doing so they would give me back the dreams that I still had for my son, though these now seemed to be just slipping through my fingers. There were days when Mark and I were unable to talk about it at all, but also days when we could talk of nothing else. 'What will we do if it is autism?' I would ask Mark. 'Listen,' Mark would say, 'let's not jump the gun. The only thing we know for sure is that he has glue ear. All we can do is to wait for the outcome. No one has actually mentioned autism. Surely it can't be autism.' This last statement was always more of a question than a statement and I didn't have an answer.

I remember clearly the Sunday before Joshua was due to go to the hospital. We were in church, and on this particular Sunday the pastor said that he felt led to pray for individuals. I asked him to pray for Joshua. He knew that Joshua had glue ear and that his appointments were imminent. He anointed his head with a little oil and prayed. To this day I can remember it all so clearly. I knew straightaway that God had touched Joshua by His Holy Spirit. As soon as the pastor started to pray he stopped wriggling furiously, became instantly still and very quiet (most unlike him). I didn't know what exactly had happened but I knew that God had met with our son. Further confirmation came the following day when I was standing at the top of the stairs. I could see Joshua at the bottom; he was just about to throw the videos from the cupboard in the hallway and decorate the floor with them again! I shouted down to him, 'Joshua, no!' I was not really expecting him to respond to me, or to turn and look, since he had his back to me. However, to my absolute amazement, he stopped and turned around and looked straight up at me. I knew then that Joshua had heard me. For a few seconds we just stared at each other and for the first time in ages I felt that he was really seeing me. So it was no great surprise when we got to the hospital and they told us that, after testing Joshua's hearing, he no longer appeared to have glue ear! However they were still very concerned because he clearly had problems. He just would not look at them and showed little response when they spoke to him. As parents we sat watching, silently willing Joshua to turn, to look when called and to respond in some way. He did not. They didn't say much but it was their silence that confirmed our fears for Joshua. It was quite apparent to us that the same alarm bells that had been going off in us, for some time now, were also resounding in their ears. We were frightened and bewildered. Joshua, on the other hand, was blissfully unaware.

We were asked to bear with them while they called in a paediatrician to observe Joshua. She also tried hard to communicate with him. Joshua of course was having none of this and gave very little eye contact to the doctor. She tried asking Joshua questions but got nowhere. The doctor then asked us all sorts of questions about him. Again it was more what was not being said that scared us. She looked solemn and pensive but gave very little away. I got the impression that she had a good idea of what was wrong with our son but she wouldn't say. She just kept saying that he no longer had a hearing problem so his behaviour couldn't be attributed to that. The paediatrician would not commit herself, even when asked directly. She suggested that Joshua be referred to another paediatrician. So although no diagnosis was given we knew that whatever was wrong with Joshua was serious. Autism was now no longer at the back of my mind and I was convinced that this was the problem.

Clouds of helplessness swept over us as we waited for yet another date. We had both hoped, against all the odds, that everything would be resolved with these appointments and that they would be able to help Joshua. We just wanted this nightmare to be over. I had hoped to take him back to nursery with some positive news but still I had none. I can't even say that life went back to normal because life was no longer normal. The lead up to Christmas was a welcomed distraction with all of the activity which surrounds that time of the year. A few days after Christmas we were sitting nervously with Joshua in the paediatrician's office. We were hoping that he would shed some light on the exact nature of the problems we were dealing with. The paediatrician was kind and tried to put us at ease as best he could. He spent a lot of time asking questions about Joshua. He wanted to know if there had been anything unusual about the pregnancy and birth. He wanted to know what he had been like as a baby and all about his developmental milestones. The questions kept coming. 'Was there anyone else in the family with similar problems?' 'What were his siblings like?' 'What sort of temperament did Joshua have?' 'How did Joshua interact with the rest of the family?' 'How did he ask for things?' The questions came thick and fast and I felt my head start to spin. Ironically, clarity seemed to come with the answer to every question and I could see, quite clearly, just how different my little one was. The doctor then spent some time trying to engage with Joshua. Again it was a very one-sided conversation, with the doctor doing most of the work and Joshua behaving as though the man wasn't even there. Once more, we silently willed Joshua to break into 'normal mode' and to do or say something positive, but he was not going to play ball and was far more interested in the toys in the room. Although Joshua interacted with us, he only ever seemed to respond to other people if he chose to. Typically that day wasn't one of those times of course. The paediatrician was taking notes the whole time. Then he stopped and we knew we had come to the point where he would give us his diagnosis. This was the moment at which our lives had the potential to change forever.

He started off by saying that he was almost inclined to sit on the fence with this one, since the referral notes showed that Joshua's hearing had been affected by severe glue ear. Also, even though Joshua ignored people most of the time he didn't always ignore us. He loved to come to us for frequent cuddles and kisses and was extremely demonstrative. He said that much of the behaviour that he was seeing could be explained away by his recent hearing problems, but they would also be what you would expect to see when a child has an autistic spectrum disorder. There, he had said it and it couldn't be unsaid. Numbness gripped my mind but surprise did not. In a way it was a relief to hear it said out loud. In direct contrast, the shreds of hope that I had held on to so tightly now lay in tatters on the floor. We sat and listened to whatever the sympathetic paediatrician said next. We nodded at the appropriate times and tried to concentrate but all the while our minds had been completely taken over by that word 'autism'. That was all I could hear echoing in my mind. At the end of the appointment we took our little Joshua home. I wanted to hold him so close and tell him over and over again how much I loved him. At the same time, I wondered if he would ever really understand what I meant. It was as though the little boy we loved had died and in his place stood an impostor.

We came to realise that in a sense we were experiencing the death of all our hopes for Joshua and his future. It was like a sort of bereavement. It was the loss of the future that we had assumed he would have that we were actually mourning. Of course as parents we can never be sure of what the future holds for any of our children, but we dare to hope and dream for them anyway. It could be a good job, marriage, a family and so on. It was beginning to dawn on us that we might have to let go of those dreams and be totally open-minded about what was in store for him. All we knew was that now it might not be as we had once hoped. We were totally unsure of what lay before us, not only for him but also for us as a family. I felt wretched inside and I know Mark did too. 'Mark,' I whispered, 'I can't believe that our worst nightmare has become reality. It hurts so much when I look at Joshua now. I just don't know how to begin accepting this.' Mark just nodded. The devastation was clearly visible on his face. I knew this must be bringing back childhood memories of his special needs brother. His next comment confirmed my suspicions. 'I feel so robbed. I lost so much of my childhood because of my brother's needs. How do I stand and watch our family walk a similar path?' There was a feeling of utter helplessness that seemed to seep into our consciousness. It was as though Joshua's developmental clock had been stopped somehow. He seemed to have gone back in time and was like a helpless baby again, so small, so vulnerable. But from what I knew about autism (which I have to say at that point was very little) vulnerability was something that he would wear like a chain around his neck and all I wanted to do was to cry until I could cry no more. Instead, I just held him and told him over and over how much I loved him. I didn't want him to see my tears, not that he would have understood them anyway. For that ignorance ironically I was glad. We drove back from the hospital in a dazed state, wanting to say so much but unable to talk out loud. Although we now officially saw Joshua as different, life for him carried on as normal. In a sense he was safe in his oblivion. We didn't have to hide anything from him or break the news to him because he was encased in this invisible bubble of 'mind blindness'. Although there seemed to be so many negatives, we now had to find a way to clutch onto the positives together. Of course the paediatrician could no more predict what lay ahead for Joshua than we could. Only God knew what the future held for our son. The paediatrician had highlighted some of the things that we ourselves knew but perhaps took for granted. He had noted that Joshua was used to having children around him and so we didn't always have to avoid busy places. This enabled him to cope with his nursery setting and the buzz of activity that went with it. He didn't seem to crave sameness and routines that much. Was that because we purposefully went out of our way to avoid him getting hooked on unnecessary routines, or was that just down to Joshua? I really didn't know. The doctor could also see that the situation was eased, in a small way, by the fact that he was demonstrative. But I guess our big question was, where exactly was our God in all of this and why would He allow it to happen? Everything seemed so unfair and so heart-breaking. I felt as though part of me was starting to shut down. Information overload perhaps. It was as though a thick layer of numbness had wrapped itself around me like a blanket. It appeared to be cushioning me from the reality of it all, preventing me from feeling the full depth of loss that would have just crushed me, on that particular day of revelation. Was that God cushioning the blow? Nevertheless there was a choice to be made; we both knew we had to consciously choose to believe that God was right there with us. Those feelings were not just going to appear because ultimately it was an issue of trust. At that point I was finding it difficult to see God in it at all and nothing seemed to make sense anymore. It was hard because there were so many emotions vying for our attention. There were days when I felt totally safe and at peace in God's presence. At other times I felt totally abandoned by Him and utterly lost which was unbearable. Yet when all was said and done, I knew that God was my backbone and that without Him I would be unable to function as I should. The days passed and when the house was empty, or if everyone had already settled down for the night, I would cry out to God. I would be totally overwhelmed by the futility of my own efforts to make things better for Joshua. The stark reality was that I could do very little. I couldn't change his diagnosis. I realised perhaps on a deeper level just how powerless I really was. Tears of total grief would then fall and I would almost double over with the pain of it all. "How could You allow us to go through this, God?" I would demand. "You say You love us but I just cannot understand or see Your love in any of this." It was normally during these dark times that

He seemed distant. I guess in my grief I was simply pushing Him away. Even so, deep down, I knew that He understood since God knows me better than I know myself. Finally when the tears had stopped flowing and there were no more to be shed, almost without warning, I would sense His gentle presence. I knew that God was still there, loving me and hurting with me. It hadn't been God who had walked away from me, but me from Him. God was still where He had always been, right by my side. No, I wouldn't ever understand why God had allowed our lives to be changed in this way but the question was simple, could I allow myself to trust Him in this? Was I prepared to trust God even when I didn't understand and when life hurt to the core? Although I was caught up in my own sorrow, I would often consider the many other families affected in a similar way because now I knew they were out there. My eyes had been opened. Now I could see them and perhaps my heart was touched with some of God's compassion. My heart went out to them and I wondered how they coped. As for myself, I was so thankful to God that Joshua was our third child. Firstly, I had spent precious time with my other children before the diagnosis. Although there would be many more precious times to come, I was somehow grateful for this. I had known a time without autism in our family. Secondly, because he had been baby number three, Joshua had to fit in with the rest of us. From very early on he had experienced the activities that his siblings were involved in, which I was sure had done him good. From just a few weeks old he attended a weekly music group with his brothers. He carried on going right up until he was four. Maybe that is why he loves music so much. If he had been our first I wonder whether he would have had such a variety of experiences. Would I have done things differently because of his problems? On the other hand if he had been the only one I may have had more time to give solely to him. Would that have made a difference? Could I have given him more? Who knows! There were so many questions.

How to communicate?
How to get through?
Who can tell me what I should do?

Hundreds of strategies
Methods galore!
My mind is awash with it all

Father navigate me through this maze
Stop me from feeling so afraid

Prevent me from drowning in this emotional sea
Give me room to breathe, to still be me.

3 FINDING OUR WAY

Of course, following Joshua's diagnosis, I was hungry for any knowledge about autism. I bought books, read articles and tried to work my way through the vast quantities of information on the internet. It was as though I had an insatiable appetite for the subject. I needed to be informed because maybe then I would understand more of what this actually meant for my son's future. I wanted to find out what we as his parents could do to help. Surely to be well informed was to be better equipped. It was especially interesting to find out about other people's experiences, whether they themselves were on the autistic spectrum or if they too had a child who was autistic.

I was struck by the fact that in most of the books that I read, it stated that autism was a life-long condition almost immediately. It sounded like a terminal illness for which there was no room for hope. It was a hard fact to swallow so soon after Joshua's diagnosis and each time it would knock the wind out of my sails. At times it was almost impossible to hold on to the positives, but cling to them I did; if I gave up then what would be the point in getting out of bed each morning? Besides what else was there to do? What choice did I have? He is my son.

As Christians we continued to look to God, always searching for answers. Sometimes they came, other times they did not and we had to wait. When we fell apart, as we often did, it was God who picked us up and dusted us down, soothing our wounds along the way. I am not suggesting for a minute that the fact that we are Christians makes it easy because it doesn't, of course. In fact in many ways it can make it harder to understand. You find yourself trying to work out why God allows these situations into your life. It is easy to be left feeling completely deserted. I guess the bottom line for us is that God is ultimately in control and wants only the best for us. Part of our journey through all of this is getting to that place of understanding and acceptance of our situation. Perhaps it is a lifelong journey. Along the way we have realised that this world is far bigger than just our little family unit and there is a much larger picture that, in its entirety, only God sees. We might have been knocked off course when we realised that Joshua had problems, but God wasn't because He already knew what was around the corner. Although my emotions were all over the place I became aware, perhaps in a new way, that it wasn't God who had changed, it was our situation. He was, as I had often read in my bible, the same before and after Joshua's diagnosis. I love my son dearly but I have come to appreciate that God loves him so much more than I can even comprehend. Slowly I was realising that I could trust God with Joshua. For me this was trust on a different level and I needed to trust God even when life stung. Was I prepared to follow God when he was leading us, as a family, to a place where I certainly would not have chosen to go and to be brutally honest where I didn't want to go? Although our concerns for Joshua were mounting I knew that it would ultimately be God's plan and not mine for

Joshua's life. I also knew that I had to depend on God for his future, even if it meant a future that was not in line with my dreams for Joshua. At times life is a bit like being out at sea, I guess. The weather and conditions can never be guaranteed. As I have felt the waves of life come crashing down around me, bitterness and anger have sometimes overtaken me and often it has been directed at God. He has listened and despite my misconceptions, His patience and His love for me have never wavered. After I have stopped ranting, calmed down, and paused to listen, I would hear him whispering ever so gently. The message was always the same: He loved me and He understood how I felt. It has been a process of being slowly stripped, of some of those things that I thought were so important to my personal happiness and that of my family. We have found ourselves heading for unfamiliar waters. It is an ever-changing route that we are going along. Maybe this is just life? We constantly have to stop, steady ourselves and catch our breath before getting up again and re-joining the race of life. We had thought we knew roughly where we were going but then we found ourselves travelling along new terrain. Acceptance is a major key in all of this and I try to accept what today brings but the door of hope is always open for tomorrow. As parents we are naturally protective of our children. When your child has special needs you may want to wrap them up in cotton wool and protect them from the world. The trouble is that ultimately they live in the real world and even if they only have limited understanding of this fact, we as parents cannot change that.

Our road of discovery continued. Joshua carried on going to nursery. There were great days and also the not so good days. In my heart I was still reaching for the stars for him. We were so grateful for the nursery that Joshua attended. His experiences there helped to encourage him to venture out of that hiding place deep down within himself. Just being at nursery did so much for him. He continued to receive the much needed one to one supervision the entire time he was there and he was encouraged to join in as much as he possibly could. The expectations put on him were very much in line with those we had at home and it worked well. Obviously, there was a certain amount of structure which Joshua had to learn to cope with. At the beginning of the session it was register time when all of the children would gather together in one room and the teacher would note who was present. Afterwards they would then perhaps sing a few songs with actions. This was definitely the most difficult time for Joshua. Each child would enter the room, sit down on a chair and then wait for the session to start. Unlike his peers, Joshua would not listen for his name. Instead of sitting down for any length of time, he preferred to wander around looking for something of greater interest to do. Nevertheless, he was encouraged to participate even if it was just for a few minutes. They would then take him out when he had clearly had enough. It took some time but eventually he became more tolerant of this part of the session.

The helpers were extremely loving and patient with him as they took turns to 'Josh watch'. They got to know him well and were usually one step ahead of him which was no mean feat! They began to comprehend what he was trying to communicate and to recognise when it was perhaps time to end an activity. He was getting the very best stimulation while he was there and I left him feeling confident that he was in capable hands. He began attending two morning sessions a week which was gradually built up to five mornings. He left home in a good frame of mind each day knowing that he was on his way to nursery. On the very odd occasion when he appeared reluctant it would generally be because he wasn't feeling well and was coming down with something. However, these times have always been few and far between and Joshua continues to be a very healthy child. Perhaps the positive side to Joshua consuming all sorts of inedible substances has resulted in a robust immune system, who knows? As well as becoming accustomed to register time there were many other activities to be tackled. Free play followed register and the children could choose from the various activities that had been put out for that day. Joshua flitted from one task to another not really settling for any one in particular. He did like painting and play doh but he still had a tendency to sneak bits of play doh into his mouth when he thought that no one was looking. Free play was followed by 'tidy up time' when the children were encouraged to help put away the toys and he too was urged to join in. Snack time was the next major item on the agenda and the children were expected to sit down at one of two tables, for a drink and a snack. A simple enough task you might think but Joshua had to learn to sit and wait. He was generally ok when he was eating, but it was waiting for the food and staying seated after he had finished that would stretch him. It was very difficult when he was not occupied. Even though he was seated with ten other children he was only really aware of his own personal needs. If he saw food on someone else's plate, that he fancied the look of, he had pretty much digested it before the person realised that it was gone. So there were lots of challenges in this seemingly simple activity that he had to begin to master.

At home, Joshua was always encouraged to stay seated throughout mealtime and not to wander off. Mealtimes in our household would be constantly interrupted with the phrase, 'Sit down Joshua!' It was high on our list of priorities because as a family we wanted to have the freedom to eat out. This might be going out for a snack, a meal or just a drink and we didn't want Joshua chasing around the place, helping himself to everyone else's food. That is exactly what he would do if left to his own devices. There has been more than one occasion when we have been in a public place; Joshua has taken himself off and started to eat some unsuspecting child's food (or adult's for that matter!). It has happened at a soft play area or at a church lunch for instance. Joshua has even been caught feasting on someone's leftovers! He really isn't that fussy; chips are chips as far as he is concerned! On one occasion when Mark took the children out for lunch Joshua managed to grab a chip from a man's plate, on the way out. I wasn't there but I could imagine exactly how Mark must have felt. Fortunately the man wasn't bothered at all and thankfully he saw the funny side of it. I suppose the point is that you can never completely relax when you take Joshua out!

Living with the strain of autism soon becomes the norm. You forget what it is like to be able to let your child go off and play, while you relax and chat to the other parents at a party or a friend's house. It can be extremely tiring because it is like having a child in permanent hyper toddler mode. We have to constantly scan the room to keep track of his whereabouts. If you go anywhere new you automatically carry out a check of the possible danger spots that must be avoided at all costs. It is not so bad at home because as far as we can we have 'Joshua proofed' our house, but not everyone has a Joshua! Most places are not set up for coping with him. Most of the time he is fine but there are always occasions when things do not go as planned, like the time Joshua decided to do some extensive pruning in a friend's flower garden! Luckily it was a close friend but I did feel so bad when I saw the huge splash of colour on the patio of severed flower heads. In the short term, it would definitely have been easier to just stop doing the things that Joshua found difficult and to concentrate on the activities that he coped well with. It would have made for an easier life for us all (for a while anyway). Looking back I think we had probably pushed through some of the barriers without even realising it, way before he was diagnosed.

It is a constant challenge when you have other children because their needs have to be met too. We don't want to accommodate Joshua's needs at the expense of theirs or vice versa. At times, it is difficult to make the call and to know when we are just expecting too much of Joshua or when we really need to push through. I guess that is just parenting! Each child is different and what works with one doesn't necessarily work with another. Also families differ in their approach and they each have their own coping strategies. There are so many factors to be taken into account, including the specific needs of the child and their personality. It also depends on the family, their personal circumstances and how much support they have.

During Joshua's time at nursery there were numerous activities that were difficult for him, due to his lack of understanding among other things. The story at the end of the session was a winding down time for the other children but not so for Joshua. It involved sitting peacefully as well as concentrating which was hard. Also it was tough for Joshua if the story did not hold any interest for him which was usually the case. After all, it would hardly be fair on everyone else if the stories were always about 'Thomas the Tank engine,' 'Rosie and Jim,' or, 'Bob the Builder,' his favourites at the time! We found that slowly, Joshua came to accept many of the activities that he had found so intolerable to begin with. Gradually his resistance to them seemed to fade and sometimes even disappear altogether. I don't think he ever got a lot out of story time but he came to accept it as part of the routine. (His developing reading skills and his greater understanding has meant that he now enjoys stories much more. He now chooses from a wider range of reading material and has been known to approach me, book in hand, requesting 'Story time.' Who would have predicted that?).

Swimming was probably one of the most dramatic turnarounds for Joshua. With absolutely no warning at all, pretty much overnight, he became a water baby who would happily spend most of his time in the pool, possibly only venturing out to eat from time to time. To this day he still loves swimming and is very confident in the water. We are not sure what changed his mind and maybe we will never know.

Although the nursery, that Joshua attended, was not

set up for children with autism they were keen to give it a go and adapt. They made sure that they had specific people to work with him. They really did their homework and made it a priority to find out as much as they could about autistic spectrum disorders. In doing so they of course were better equipped to help him. The channels of communication were very much open; when I picked him up they always had time to tell me about his morning and how he had been.

There is a wealth of information out there about autism and it is easy to get swamped with the enormity of it all. In addition to this, there is an abundance of advice to be had from various professionals. It can be quite overwhelming to say the least. However, as parents, we have had to remember that there is still no one who knows our child the way that we do and sometimes you just have to go with your gut feelings. We certainly didn't know for sure which nursery setting would work for Joshua, but we went with what we thought would suit him best at that time. Some people opt for a special needs nursery while others might choose home education. Each child's needs are different and parents usually have an idea of what would suit their child best. We only really knew our child's strengths and weaknesses and for him a mainstream setting worked well. Very gradually it gently teased him out of the solitary world that he was in, long enough to allow him to take a peek at what was happening beyond his comfort zone. Slowly he became a bit more interested in other people and at times could interact for long enough to enjoy the experience. Well at least that was how it appeared to us. We would see flickers of hope when he did something for the first time or if he joined in with an activity, even if it was just for a while.

Joshua was becoming more accustomed to changes in routine. Often progress was made as a result of us just simply getting on with living. It wasn't always the result of a conscious effort. Being a younger sibling he often got taken along to parties, friend's houses, fairgrounds and the like. Surely these experiences have helped, in small ways, to acclimatize him to this startling, busy and unpredictable world in which we live? Who can really know for sure? Would Joshua have been the 'water baby' that he is today if he had been my first? Would I have been quite so determined to press through his fear of swimming when his shouting pierced through the fun and laughter around him? If it had been only him, and there were not three others keen to get into the water, would I have reacted differently? I will never know the answers to those questions.

His nursery experiences may have been a bit like spending time in a super-sized family with lots of faces, activity and noise. Well whatever the reason it was definitely a turning point in Joshua's life and this was positive for us all. Several people were now involved in helping Joshua to move forward. The paediatrician, who had initially diagnosed Joshua, had passed his name to the various services responsible for helping children with special needs. In time we were contacted by the special needs co-ordinator (senco) for our area, who arranged to visit Joshua at home. We had a long chat and during our time with her she got to know a bit about our journey with Joshua so far. It gave her a chance to get to know him and of course to assess his needs and ours as a family. She also arranged a date to observe him in his nursery setting since she was there to support the nursery too. Once she had been to the nursery, she put them in touch with an Autism Outreach Service which in turn arranged for someone, from their organisation, to also visit Joshua.

The day that Joshua was initially assessed by the Autism Outreach Service is one that I don't think I will ever forget. Yes of course, by now I knew that my son was diagnosed as being on the autistic spectrum and we were just starting to decode what that actually meant for Joshua and us as a family. This time was different though because the person assessing Joshua was a professional within the field. We knew that he would spend some time observing Joshua at nursery and then he would feed back to the staff. This first visit was really just to see roughly where Joshua was on the spectrum. I remember well reading a copy of the notes that he had taken during his observations. For some reason, each phrase was like an unexpected slap in the face …'there was absolutely no doubt as to the diagnosis, Joshua presented as quite severely autistic'. My heart seemed to miss a beat. It was as though each syllable of every word on that report stung me. He continued, 'My observations of Joshua lead me to conclude that a diagnosis of autism spectrum disorder would indeed be appropriate. He demonstrates significant impairments in communication skills, and social interaction and awareness. Although I did not observe unusual perseveration/obsessive tendencies during this session, I understand that these are also evident in his behaviour'. The same tell-tale signs that had caught our attention were noted in his observations: 'During registration, Joshua paid no attention to others and to the whole-group activity; he did not look at other children or adults (except fleetingly at the adult with him when repeatedly prompted)'. 'In the free play session he exhibited the same patterns of behaviour. He showed no interest in and did not communicate in any way with other children or adults, but looked around constantly at the objects set out around the room. He did not seem perturbed in any way by the presence of other children, but behaved as though they were not there.' 'Attempts at communication with Joshua were difficult because of his constant movement.' His observations were followed by several recommendations and strategies. The eloquence with which he was able to summarise my son's long list of problems was delivered with great sensitivity but still I smarted from the fresh pain and shock. For some reason it was like receiving the diagnosis all over again. I was normally quite strong and optimistic but not so on that day. Of course I already knew that Joshua had problems, but maybe it was at this precise point that the information moved from my head down to my heart and oh it hurt so much. I wanted to scream out loud but I managed to hold it together as I read on. The nursery had been told that there really was 'not a moment to waste if we wanted Joshua to reach his full potential'. There was a real sense of urgency in his remarks. Waves of grief just kept washing over me again and again and I felt suffocated by the bleakness of it all.

Joshua and I wandered out of nursery to join Mark, who had waited in the car. I got into the car with Joshua but felt that I just could not dump all of my despair onto Mark. So I didn't tell him how I was feeling but just gave him the cold hard facts. Both

Mark and I were pretty much in the same place emotionally and neither of us felt like going home, where all we would do was to focus on our situation. So instead we popped in to see a friend on the way home. She will never really know how she managed to lift our spirits that day. I believe that God's love was flowing through her to us. She was excited to see us because she had dreamt about Joshua a few nights back and was eager to share her dream with us. In her dream Joshua was older and had developed in so many ways. 'He was able to communicate his needs,' she said 'and I was actually able to communicate with Joshua because his speech was more developed.' She also recalled that 'Joshua was happier and more content in himself. He was much more a part of what was going on around him.' She encouraged us to keep going. Somehow everything that we needed to hear came from her that day. Perhaps it was because she has had experience of working with people with special needs, I don't know. Well whatever the reason, we both left feeling uplifted and were able to once again hold on to the positives. So, armed with a more optimistic disposition, I did as the nursery had asked and contacted the Autism Outreach Service when I got home.

As I had been led to believe, the man who had assessed Joshua was eager to do what he could to help. He planned to return to the nursery soon and advise them on the best way forward. He was keen for us all to work together to achieve one essential goal which was ultimately to help Joshua. The group of people who were now involved with Joshua's well-being was growing. The area senco, the representative from the autism outreach service, the nursery leader and two nursery sencos would get together with us to work out what the best way forward was. Targets and goals were set for him on a term by term basis. In addition to this it had been decided that Joshua should be taken into a quiet, distraction free, room where he could be encouraged to communicate and to learn through play, on a one to one basis. This would only be for a short time during each session. Various activities were put into place to encourage better eye contact, better communication and more social interaction. Joshua was encouraged to give eye contact in order to receive a desired object. Another goal was for him to give eye contact in response to his name or to the request 'Look at me'. He was asked to copy simple physical actions, for example 'clap your hands', 'touch your nose', as well as imitating basic speech sounds. Sometimes this would be achieved through action songs and rhymes. Communication and expressive language skills were encouraged by asking Joshua to point to a desired real object in response to the question, 'What do you want?' He was also expected to match real objects to photographs of the items. Simple activities such as puzzles, picture lotto and building blocks were used to make these sessions fun. The results were recorded and built on. He rose to the challenge and progressed well through his various tasks. Occasionally another child would join Joshua, the idea being to encourage Joshua to 'play'.

Life is full of first experiences and it was at nursery that Joshua had his first taste of being involved in the Christmas play. I can't tell you how lovely it was to see him sitting on the stage all dressed up with his helper. Joshua was now four years old. Admittedly he didn't do a lot and wasn't always that aware of the entire goings on, but he was there and would occasionally even attempt to join in with the singing. Back then the goal was really for Joshua to stay sitting with the other children on the stage, without making too much of a fuss. The person in charge of the Christmas production was none other than the lady who had run the music group that Joshua had attended and so she was familiar with him. With the passing of each play (Christmas or Easter) we would see improvements. They may not have always been huge strides but sometimes, out of the blue, those big strides would catch you unaware and almost take your breath away. At those moments you simply wanted to tell the world. During the two years that he attended nursery he changed so much. I almost wished that he could stay for another year, but time had raced ahead again; he was nearly five and due to start school.

As well as attending nursery, Joshua also went to another play-group called 'Play and Say'. It was a small group of children and their mothers who met once a week, a bit like a small version of nursery. It was run by the area senco and a small team which included Joshua's speech therapist. The group was specifically for children who had impaired communication and developmental delays. It was a less overwhelming environment than nursery where each child would be gently encouraged to overcome their fears. They would start each session with a welcome song where the children had the opportunity to introduce themselves, if they were brave enough. Activities would follow. These would be different each week and would range from potato printing to parachute games. It was possible to have a wide range of activities due to the small number of children. Through play they were being encouraged to step out of their comfort zone into areas which they would normally avoid. Some of the children hated messy play. They tended to steer away from the craft activities or the water play and stick with what they were comfortable doing. It was a real privilege to see those very same children stepping out into an area that had once been a no go zone for them and actually getting pleasure from doing so. In the middle of the session there would be snack time. Again for some of the children it was just hard for them to join the others at the table. Different ones had to be gently coaxed into requesting a food item. Lots of encouragement and praise was always given. Each child would spend a short while with the speech therapist. It also provided the senco with a regular opportunity to touch base with the parent and to find out how things were going, or if there were any specific needs. Joshua started attending the group shortly after he was diagnosed by the paediatrician and carried on right up until he started school. I think we both benefited from the experience.

4 LIFE IS A ROLLER COASTER

Starting school is a momentous occasion for any child. It is a time of adjustment for both parent and child. However for Joshua, with all of his problems, I felt it was all of that and more. Nursery had been such a positive experience and I thought that it would be a tall order to find a school with as much to offer. Our other two boys went to a small independent Christian school, about 20 miles away from where we lived. It had been set up some 25 years ago by our group of churches. Up until Joshua's difficulties became apparent, it had been a foregone conclusion that he would also go there. However as great as it was, the school was quite small and not really set up to deal with Joshua's needs. If he were to attend he would need a lot of extra help, such as speech therapy, one to one supervision and so on. Since it was an independent school it fell outside the jurisdiction of the local education authority, whose provision did not extend to such schools. Lots of possibilities crossed our minds. Maybe he could attend the same school as his siblings albeit with lots of help, in which we could be involved in some way? The idea of home schooling him was also something else we considered, but we were concerned that he would be lacking in social stimulation. Would it be like taking a step backwards? Of course, he didn't respond in the same way that a normal child responded to his peers anyway but, nevertheless, he was still affected by what was happening around him.

We had heard about a special school, not far from the school his brothers attended, and we decided to visit. Logistically it made perfect sense for him to go there. I guess I had jumped ahead of myself and assumed it had to be the right place for him. It was indeed a good school with a team of dedicated staff. Joshua would have been in quite a small class with a couple of classroom assistants. It was also fairly new with great facilities, including a brand new swimming pool. That would definitely be a big positive for Joshua. (Also, on the same site was a primary school which catered for children without special needs. This set up presented the possibility for a certain amount of integration between the two schools, if it was considered appropriate for the child.) We were privileged to meet some of the gorgeous 'special' children who between them had a variety of needs: Downs's syndrome, Tourette's, cerebral palsy, autism and so on. I remember hearing the little boy who had Tourette's shout 'Shut up' and I don't think I will ever forget the little girl with cerebral palsy, who could do nothing but lie in her specially adapted buggy. She couldn't move and her body was completely motionless but she had the most dazzling smile. Her body may have given up but her mind was very alert and she was eager to see who the visitors were. I wondered how much attention she received from her peers. I also wondered if this would be a stimulating environment for Joshua. He was busy scanning the room and had seen that there were books in the corner. He boldly helped himself to one and started to leaf through the pages. The school was impressive so why was I disappointed? Neither Mark nor I knew why but we both felt that this was not where Joshua was meant to be. Was it because at nursery Joshua was getting one to one support and teaching and that this was something he would not get at the special school? That may have been part of it but certainly not the only reason. We prayed about it and actually visited the school again but still our gut feeling was that this was not the place. So if this was not the right school then 'where God?' we prayed. We knew that through his home life and his schooling Joshua was being encouraged to acknowledge and to be a part of our world (as much as he was able to) and not the little world that he would probably disappear into completely, if he was allowed. Nothing was ever going to change the fact that, whether he liked it or not, he lived in our world with all its hustle and bustle, its smells, its sounds and millions and billions of people. I couldn't shield or hide him from it even if I wanted to. We saw part of our role as protector, shielding him from danger and in a sense providing him with a safe haven where he could escape when he needed to. Our role was also to equip him in whatever way we could and give him room to reach his full potential (whatever that might be). No, we couldn't change who Joshua was and eliminate his problems, so that he would be 'normal' and fit in. On the other hand, neither were we able to change the world around him to make sure it always accommodated him and all of his idiosyncrasies. So we were back to the drawing board as far as finding a school for Joshua was concerned. To complicate things further, we were planning to move and had our house on the market. We tried another special school but it didn't seem to suit Joshua either. The senco suggested a couple of mainstream schools that were really close to where we still lived. A mainstream school was not something that we had even contemplated but we were open to suggestions and so we arranged an appointment to see the first one.

Prior to the appointment we were both feeling unsure. 'It all seems a bit pointless visiting this school when we are planning to move. Also, I don't know how Joshua could possibly cope full time at a mainstream school. Full time school is very different to nursery,' I said to Mark. He looked thoughtful, 'Well, it won't hurt to visit although I'm not too hopeful either. But as the senco said Joshua almost needs something between special needs and mainstream.' I could hear the weariness in his voice. We were both so very tired. We visited the school, a few days later, with Joshua so that they could meet him and see what he was like for themselves. Neither of us had high expectations but as the meeting progressed we both felt surprisingly optimistic. The school senco and the head teacher were very positive. Logistically it made little sense because (although it was on our doorstep) we were looking to move away. In our hearts, however, it just felt right and we both thought that this was where God wanted Joshua to be at that time. By the end of the meeting we were all in agreement that it would be a good placement for Joshua, as long as adequate funding could be secured for the one to one support that he would need. It was decided that a gradual transition into full time education would work best for him. Joshua would attend the setting for five mornings a week initially. He was already used to this with nursery. His time there would be increased slowly until eventually he would be full time. The shift towards him attending school full time would be very much dictated by how well he was coping. Ultimately it was a case of seeing whether the placement suited Joshua. If it didn't work out then we would all have to think again. It was true that there were other special needs children at the school, including a few children who were somewhere on the autistic spectrum. However they had never had someone quite like Joshua before. So for them and for us it was a bit like venturing into the unknown. The great thing was that they were willing to look ahead, to see what needed to be put in place and to get everything sorted out as soon as possible. They contacted his nursery, set up dates for them to visit Joshua there to observe him and to get to know him. They were pleasantly surprised at how friendly and happy he seemed. They also came to see him at home which was useful. During these visits we got to know them a bit more and we just had a real peace about him going to this school. We had prayed about it a lot and visited various places. In the end God had opened a door right on our doorstep. Sometimes you just get a positive feeling about a certain place as well as the staff and you have to go with your gut feeling. It was going to be a time of much change. Not only was Joshua starting a new school but Joshua's sister was also due to start nursery. We were not sure where to send her. Ideally, I would have wanted her to attend the nursery Joshua was about to leave, but it would have resulted in our children going in three different directions which wasn't feasible! As it turned out, Megan was offered a nursery place at Joshua's new school even though she wasn't on the waiting list. Things were beginning to fall into place and I could see God's hand at work in it all. I was sad that

Joshua's time at nursery was coming to an end because he had enjoyed it there, but life is forever changing and it was time for Joshua to move on. We just had to trust God in this next step for him.

Our house sold shortly before Joshua was due to leave nursery. Our buyers were in a hurry and as we didn't want to lose the sale we decided to rent somewhere, until we found something suitable to buy. We knew that we would be moving again shortly so we wanted to make our time in rented accommodation as enjoyable as we could for us all. It was spring and the chances were we would spend the summer holidays there, so it would be more like a holiday home. It also had to be somewhere where Joshua would be quite safe if he managed to escape. Again God just provided. We found this amazing cottage in the middle of nowhere, over a mile away from a little village. It had a large garden and the setting was just perfect for us. We had already bought Joshua an outdoor trampoline for his last birthday and so we decided to buy an outdoor activity centre with swings, a slide, a seesaw etc. We hoped that with all the attractions in the garden he wouldn't feel the need to wander off, as he was in the habit of doing.

This period in our lives was a very special one. To this day I can still remember exactly how I felt the day we moved into the cottage. Mark had gone to return the removal truck, the children were with their grandparents and I was at the cottage on my own before going to join them. It was beautifully sunny even though it had been raining earlier. I was surrounded by green fields and apart from our cottage there wasn't another dwelling in sight. We had never ever lived in a place as remote as this before but it had always been a dream of ours and we were looking for a similar type of place to buy. The plan was for us and the grandparents (who also had their house on the market) to buy a large property together and then to extend. We were looking for somewhere with enough space for two self-contained dwellings. That way we hoped it would be possible to still run our own business and get the children to their schools which would now be 23 miles apart! I felt a peace that I had not felt for some time. It could easily have been just me in the world that day. All of life's busyness and strife seemed to be elsewhere. It was as though I was encapsulated in a bubble of tranquillity. What a place to spend the summer I thought as I silently thanked God. On our first visit to the cottage, contracts hadn't been exchanged on the sale of our house. The letting agents advised us that they couldn't hold it for us, as there were other people interested. However, when contracts had eventually been exchanged we tentatively enquired as to whether the cottage was still available. It turned out that it was and that, despite what we had been told, the letting agents had in fact kept it for us. So before I went to join everyone else I stood and soaked in the beauty of my surroundings and God's presence in it all. Surely Joshua would have less reason to escape in an environment such as this one, I thought. After all we were surrounded by fields and there really wasn't anywhere to escape to.

My mind quickly wandered back to the very first time Joshua had escaped. He must have been about two and a half years old at the time and we were at a friend's house. It was a gorgeous day and everyone was in the garden. Both of our families had children and there was a lot of activity. Nobody noticed that Joshua had slipped away. To this day we don't know why he went. He was not to be found anywhere in the house or garden. Then to our horror we saw that the garden gate was ajar and we knew then that he must have wandered out onto the street. We raced to the front of the house but there was simply no sign of him. Looking straight ahead, I could see the little pathway that we took each week to go to our music group. The pathway itself was quite short but it led to a very busy main road and at that moment I felt sick. Somehow I just knew that was where he had gone. I started to run towards the main road, all the while, battling to clear my mind of all the unwanted scenarios clamouring to get in. In the distance I caught sight of a couple coming towards me and I could see that they had a little child with them. My heart was racing and I strained to see the child's face. It looked like Joshua but the child was still too far away for me to be sure. My heart was like an internal clock, each beat pounding against my chest. 'Please God, please God let it be Joshua!' I pleaded silently. As he got closer I could see that it was definitely Joshua and I ran towards him frantically. After I had claimed him and thanked them over and over they told me what had happened. Apparently, just as I had feared, Joshua had headed straight for the main road and was going to cross it when they found him. They had been about to call the police. Joshua showed absolutely no signs that he was aware of the danger that he had put himself in. He wasn't at all bothered that he was away from his family or that he was with two total strangers. That feeling of dread stayed with me for some time. How could I have possibly known that it was something we would have to face again and again!

There are times when life can make you feel as though you are travelling through it on a roller coaster because there are so many unexpected twists and turns. One minute you are soaring high and the next moment you may feel as though you are heading for the ground, head first from a great height. The direction of your course is forever changing, or is that just the way it feels? Joshua's journey through school was a time of us letting go of the old and moving forward. There was no room for preconceived ideas and no trying to outguess God as to what each day, week or term held for him. It was a time to try to surrender Joshua into God's hands. Saying it is definitely the easy part; putting it into practice is always much harder. Starting school can be both daunting and exciting at the same time. For parents it is also a learning curve as we too travel alongside our children, through the educational system. We watch as they gingerly take their first few steps into this new world. We observe as they make new friends and grow accustomed to their new surroundings. We stand back to give them room to grow in confidence and stature and we proudly look on. We are there to help them and guide them. As their parents it is our role to work in partnership with the school and do our best to nurture, teach and stick on yet another plaster. We hope that in time we will reap the reward as they grow and mature, gradually becoming more independent. It is truly amazing to watch and it seems to go by so quickly. How easy it is to assume that all of these things will just naturally happen. That is after all the normal pattern of events isn't it? It is only when we come across a glitch and things don't go quite as expected, for whatever reason, that we may pause to examine the process a bit more closely. With Joshua it has often seemed as if time has stood still. It was as though, in lots of ways, his development was being played out in slow motion and every now and then (in certain areas) the pause or the stop button had been pressed.

As difficult as it is sometimes, we have to live for now and not tomorrow. When we first started out on this road it was tempting to opt out of the present and live somewhere in amongst our future hopes; a place where we wanted to be rather than where we actually were. Perhaps it was a future where Joshua would somehow wake up out of his autism and start to develop normally. Then we could step out from where we had found ourselves and get on with the life that we thought we were supposed to be living. Circumstances can be so difficult and painful at times that, it may seem, the only way forward is to try and focus on how you would like things to work out and not face them as they actually are. It is good to stay positive but sometimes life just doesn't play out as you imagined it would. Even with the best will in the world, try as we might, there appears to be only one way ahead in some situations and that is right through the centre of it. We have learnt first-hand that God is there with us. He may not always rid us of every difficulty in our lives but he has all that we need to keep going. Since God is there with us, in the midst of our pain and disappointment, we are learning that it is possible to focus on Him in it, rather than solely on our troubles. It is not always easy to do but we are learning that it is possible. Of course, we are always hopeful for the future because we can never know what surprises are waiting for us around the corner. However we still try to be mindful of where we are right now, so that we don't miss out on those blessings that are right on our doorstep.

There have been so many practical ways in which God has provided for Joshua. His transition from nursery to school was made so much easier with a teacher and a teacher's assistant (TA) who really connected with him. He seemed to take to them quickly and it was obvious that he enjoyed going to school. During Joshua's first year at school, he was allowed to spend some time in the nursery so that he could just relax and play. Occasionally they would allow another child, from his class, to go with him which worked well. Of course I wondered what the other children would make of this quirky boy with his strange ways. As it turned out I needn't have worried because they seemed to accept him for who he was quirky behaviour and all. Are children more accepting than we are as adults? Who knows? Of course it did take time for some of the children to become accustomed to Joshua, but even those who were understandably wary soon warmed. I suppose he was a bit of a novelty as far as they were concerned. His presence seemed to draw out a real nurturing instinct in the children and they just wanted to look after him. All in all it was a smooth transition from nursery to school. We were kept up to date regarding his daily activities and so we knew what he had been up to. When problems or difficulties arose they were quickly resolved. Joshua seemed to settle far more quickly than any of us had dared to hope and above all he was happy. The acceptance from the children in his class helped to make Joshua feel at home. However, there was one little girl in particular who was so kind to Joshua. He absolutely adored her and would frequently give her cuddles. Hers was the first name that he recognised and I remember him beaming as he greeted her. Hers was the first school birthday party that he was invited to. This was something that I had never thought would happen for him. It was just another indication of how gracious a group of kids they were. I suppose they were learning first hand that not everyone is the same and that being different is not always something to be scared of.

Of course it wasn't all plain sailing and there were numerous hurdles along the way. Joshua was generally a fairly placid child but there were still times when he would become frustrated, for one reason or another. He would be unable to communicate the cause of his distress and he might then resort to throwing something on the floor, hit his head or even hit out at one of the other kids. He simply didn't have the words to say that he was tired, finding a task difficult or, that he had just had enough and needed some space. There was also the fact that Joshua's concentration span was really short and even sitting for an activity, for any length of time, was hard for him. It is not unusual for children to fidget in assembly, or to find it hard to stay on task, especially when they are very young. However with maturity it is supposed to get easier. If concentration and silence were required, Joshua obviously stood out like a sore thumb.

On one occasion, the whole school was gathered together for an assembly and Joshua had been sitting fairly peacefully. Soon everyone was singing a song.

When they had finished the children sat down and Joshua decided that this was the perfect opportunity to sing a bit of a solo. He waited until all were seated and it was absolutely quiet. He then jumped up sang a line of the song loudly and sat down again, much to the amusement of everyone in the hall. I must admit I did laugh when his helper told me but I was so relieved that I hadn't been there! Even I would have gone a very deep shade of red!

Towards the end of his first year, it was decided that we needed to try and gradually increase his time at school. He began by staying in school for the whole day on a Monday and he would take a packed lunch. I felt nervous about this as he hadn't done a whole day anywhere before. It was a huge milestone for him to be staying at school with lunch box in tow. However Joshua took it all in his stride. It didn't seem to faze him at all. When it looked as though he seemed to be coping well with the introduction of a whole school day, a second full day was introduced. By the end of his first school year he was doing three full days and two half days. Again Joshua had far exceeded everyone's expectations. He had settled, seemed to be learning new things all the time and was adapting well. Yes there were difficulties. There were days when he wouldn't settle or cooperate. There would be the odd day when the people who normally looked after him couldn't be there for one reason or another. This didn't happen often. The school had accommodated for this by allowing Joshua to become familiar with a group of staff. On those occasions, when his normal helpers were not available, he was still with someone familiar. I guess after a while, the teachers and pupils became more and more used to Joshua as he did to them. I think that there is always a certain amount of adjustment needed when you have a child who is so obviously different from his peers. It is not as noticeable at home. However, when standing outside the school gates, with other parents and children, those differences seem to be up there in neon lights for all to see and scrutinise. The thing with Joshua is that he looks so normal but then he will open his mouth and all sorts of incomprehensible vocalisations come out. You then see people around you looking at him and silently wondering 'what exactly is wrong with that child?' Stoicism grows within you and you have to develop a tough outer skin and sometimes try and put yourself in their shoes. What would you be thinking if it were someone else's child and you had probably never encountered autism before? Even if you didn't actually stare, inwardly you might be tempted to. People are not necessarily being rude; they simply do not know and they are naturally curious. I have never known a time when being different doesn't attract attention of some kind. Surely this is just human nature? I really didn't know very many of the other parents because Joshua hadn't gone to the school nursery. Also, even if he had done so he wouldn't have got to know the other children socially. So you are pretty much set apart from the beginning really but it is something that has to be accepted. Again and again I have asked myself 'Would it have been harder if Joshua had been my only child and this was all I knew?' I still don't know. The experience was completely different when I went to pick up his brothers and sister because they interacted with their peers, on a social level that Joshua wasn't even aware of.

So, eventually Joshua was full time at school and was still getting a lot out of the experience. He seemed to adjust to new situations and people very quickly and when there were changes to his working day, he was generally able to cope. Although he was taking only small steps forward it was rewarding nonetheless. He would sit at his work station and complete the various tasks that were given to him. He learnt to write his name and would get excited if he saw it written down on a label, or a book for instance. He clearly recognised it as being his name. We were impressed when he started to learn to read. It was truly amazing to hear him since it was something that I could never have imagined. Initially, I think it was more a case of him learning to read by memory rather than phonetically, but we were not complaining. It was a start! As Joshua became more familiar with his letters, he was soon attempting to sound out the beginnings of words. This showed that he was starting to associate the individual letters with their specific sound and trying to read phonetically. In spite of this, he did seem to have limited comprehension of the text he was reading. So various activities and matching games were used to try and develop his understanding. Joshua was encouraged to spell words with letter tiles. He then went on to construct simple sentences using pictures and words. He benefited from various computer programs and with time his understanding grew. He was still limited in his speech and was way behind his peers but all in all he was making progress. Joshua's development was a series of miniscule steps. It wasn't just a case of achieving academically but more importantly he needed life skills behind him. He needed to be taught how to socialise and being in an ordinary state school was teaching him aspects of this.

It was amazing to see Joshua being invited to lots of birthday parties. It has to be said though that, on these occasions, he did need to be watched like a hawk. Left to his own devices he would make his way over to the birthday cake and simply help himself! There were a couple of times when he nearly got there and at one party he did actually manage to sneak a tiny piece of icing. I felt terrible and apologised over and over. Understanding is something that we take for granted. Joshua still didn't fully realise that he shouldn't touch the birthday cake or the presents, even if he could reach them. Neither could he comprehend how the host would feel if he were allowed to do these things. Party games didn't come naturally either and he needed to be shown how to play them. Some of them he could be a part of while others simply involved me playing for him, with him being the puppet and me playing the puppeteer. The main thing was that he was for the most part enjoying himself and developing new life skills along the way. It was incredibly hard work and it would have been easier to just not bother but gradually it became less of a chore. Slowly Joshua began to learn what was expected of him. We have come to realise that just because Joshua learns to do something, it doesn't necessarily mean that he understands exactly why he has to do it. He doesn't empathise with or relate to others as a normally functioning child would. He may learn not to touch the birthday cake or not to take food from other people's plates, but it isn't necessarily because he can understand how the person, on the receiving end, might feel. He is not motivated by the feelings of others and I am unsure as to how much he comprehends in the whole complex area of the emotions. Nevertheless we are continually striving to push through these situations in the hope that eventually the penny will drop (even if just partially and not completely).

Some parties were easier than others. If there was a bouncy castle then Joshua would be in his element and would spend most of his time on it. He even enjoyed disco parties because he could dance around and watch all of the lights bouncing off the walls. It was more difficult for him if it involved a party entertainer for example. He didn't understand the humour and he would lose interest quickly. It then became almost impossible to keep him seated. Sometimes I would take a few snacks in my bag that he could eat while waiting. If it got too much I would have to take him out. Although it was tiring, I was motivated by the fact that Joshua was making progress. He was starting to understand why people had parties and he had begun associating certain things with parties such as cake, candles, presents and the like. He would get really excited when he was told that he was off to a party. It was therefore a momentous occasion when all of his party going started to pay off. Joshua was now in his second or third year at school and he had been to quite a few parties. At this particular one there was an entertainer and the children were all sitting down on the floor watching. For me personally it was one of those times when you just want to shout out 'eureka' from a great height. This was the first time that Joshua didn't need me to sit with him. Instead I was with some of the other mums where I could still see him. He was sitting on the floor in between two of his classmates. They were showing him what to do and he was following their cue. That was not his sole accomplishment. Temptation in the form of a table full of party food was just across the room and I could see him glancing over every now and then. If his gaze seemed to linger, a little too long, I would make a point of catching his eye and mouthing, 'Not yet, food later,' while shaking my head. That seemed to satisfy him. You see at long last he was beginning to comprehend what 'later' actually meant and so he understood that at a certain time he would actually be allowed some food. This was a major milestone for him. Through going to all of these parties he was learning and practising social skills and I could not have been more proud that day.

5 AVOIDING THE POTHOLES

The concept of sharing and small children does not naturally go hand in hand. Throw in a splash of autism and things are further complicated due to a genuine lack of awareness and reasoning. For Joshua, learning to share is still an on-going process. You don't realise how important it is to grasp the necessity of sharing until you have a child who just doesn't get it. Often trying to teach Joshua is like trying to communicate to him in a foreign language. Going to the park is something most children love to do (Joshua included). It is all about negotiating through play and it involves taking turns which requires waiting and sharing. Joshua loves to go to the park and would quite happily push obliviously past every child in his way, if he were allowed to. He has had to learn what acceptable behaviour is and what is unacceptable. These social rules, that we often take for granted, are not naturally part of Joshua's make up and he continually struggles to make sense of them. For him the best way to learn these life skills is literally to practise them over and over. He still has a long way to go but has done amazingly well and enjoys parks, bouncy castles, soft play areas, fun fairs and so much more. We are constantly trying to minimize the limitations and stress that his difficulties cause him. We want him to have as free a life as possible and to be as fulfilled as he can be. There have been lots of situations which would have been easier to avoid for a less complicated and quieter life, in the short term, but we try and think about the long term goals. Let's be real about it though, it certainly is not always possible to push through. We are only human, with a limited supply of energy. There will always be those times when you just don't have what it takes to keep going. We have learnt that it is ok and sometimes necessary to miss an activity and to have a quiet day, in order to recharge our batteries. It all helps to keep you going in the long run I'm sure. There are certain events that we simply choose to miss out on because the effort spent will far outweigh what any of us will get out of it. Other times we may just get to that point when we are just too tired to battle on and so we do what is right for us as a family, not what is perhaps expected of us. To be honest some of the time we are pressured by our own expectations as well as external ones. There are other instances when we feel it necessary to have Joshua looked after for a few hours. We are then able to concentrate solely on our other children. Constantly having to press through different events is tiring. It just wasn't (and still isn't) possible to tackle everything all at once. It wouldn't have been fair on us or on Joshua. Also, he naturally has his likes and dislikes, as do each of us. We have had to accept that there are things that he may never master and that is ok. It isn't for us to set the limits in Joshua's life. We are learning to accept that as God's domain.

Toilet training was definitely an uphill battle. Having gone through the process with two boys already I thought I knew enough to survive it with Joshua. How naïve I was! As it turned out Joshua's little sister was out of nappies before he was!

Admittedly it was a very speedy affair with her but, having said that, it was still not what I was expecting. I remember well the summer during which we were determined to toilet train Joshua. Perhaps we should have consulted Joshua first because he, on the other hand, was adamant that he was not going to be made to use the toilet. We had been through all of this before with our other children and we thought we had a plan. Really, how hard could it be! So we organised ourselves and took turns to keep an eye on him. Joshua was put on the toilet regularly. However the moment you took your eyes off him there would simply be a puddle on the floor! Our plans for toilet training Joshua rapidly went downhill when he started to go through a phase of smearing! The whole room would have to be disinfected and he would have to be scrubbed from head to toe. The many times that we would go and check on Joshua just before we were about to go to bed and discover that there was mess everywhere (and I mean everywhere) was simply disheartening. Of course by that time Joshua would have fallen asleep. He would then have to be woken up and the long drawn out cleaning ritual would begin. It was totally demoralizing. So at the end of the holidays he was still in nappies. We had tried every trick and technique in the book, and more, and had no results to show for it. Our health visitor arranged for an incontinence advisor to visit who told us that this was a common problem among autistic children. She added that there were lots of children, much older than Joshua, who were still struggling in this area. She arranged for us to get a regular supply of nappies until they were no longer needed, advised us to carry on doing what we were doing and not to lose heart because it would happen eventually. I found it all quite depressing but knew that she was talking from experience. We were told that it might simply be that the control was not there yet and he was just not ready. She insisted that he would get there in the end. Most importantly we tried not to let it become a battleground because we knew that this would only serve to make things far worse. We left it for a while and then tried again bracing ourselves. Joshua of course had the last laugh and surprised us all by becoming dry within the week. He was finally wearing pants and using the toilet to wee. We were only half way there but we had moved on. It meant that he could go to school in pants and use the toilet there. He also overcame his fear of noisy hand dryers which was useful since they are in most public toilets these days. We made a point of taking him to as many different toilets as we could so that he didn't become obsessive about having to use a particular one. It was quite a while later before Joshua would do anything other than wee in the toilet. It was a long time in coming but again it was when he was ready. Of course like most children, he had accidents but eventually he could be taken anywhere and he would often ask to use the toilet. He got there in the end!

All of these 'battles' have caused me to stop and think about the ordinary, run of the mill, life experiences that we go through. It is usually only when they present a problem that we even dwell on them at all. For Joshua most of these normal things like visits to the dentist or to the hairdressers were both challenging for him and for us! To watch Joshua having his hair cut was indeed a sorry sight. He would scream and struggle all the way through it. After a while we realised that it was the clippers that he was most frightened of. Even though his hair was scissor cut he was very aware of other people who were having their hair cut using the clippers, including his brothers. Was it a reaction to that particular noise or indeed sensory overload that he was experiencing? We don't know for sure, but it may well have been. After several visits Joshua seemed to realise that if they were not being used on him he would be ok and he started to calm down a bit. He still didn't like going to the hairdressers but he had begun to tolerate it. Was this anything to do with the reward of a lolly pop at the end I wonder? Then the breakthrough came! On one particular visit he was just not bothered about the clippers being used at all and he was as good as gold. In fact he was so compliant that he was like a different child. We were not sure why but we were encouraged to keep pressing on and were so pleased with him. Sometime later Mark decided to cut his brother's hair at home because we couldn't get an appointment, before the school term started. Joshua wandered into the kitchen with a look of fascination on his face. He watched with interest while clumps of hair fell to the floor. As soon as Mark had finished Joshua sat himself down, in the hot seat, so that Mark could do the same to his hair (which didn't actually need cutting). We all watched in amazement as Mark pretended to use the clippers on Joshua's hair. However Joshua was not going to have the wool pulled over his eyes and he could see that none of his hair had fallen to the ground. He was not about to move until Mark had actually used the clippers on his hair. Only then did he get up. We were surprised but thought that Joshua was more than satisfied with his mini haircut. While we were all downstairs marvelling at Joshua's latest achievement he sneaked upstairs. He sought out a pair of scissors and then proceeded to give himself the most atrocious haircut of all time! I could not believe it when I saw him. His hair was simply a jagged mess. He looked absolutely awful and hilarious at the same time and I could not help but laugh. I am not sure how long he had been cutting it for but he had cut ridges, in his hair, all over the top of his head! Of course the only way we could make him look anywhere near presentable was to cut his hair really short which would involve using the clippers. Is this what he had in mind I wonder? I suspect so! If so, he definitely got his wish! He clearly enjoyed the experience so much that, whenever he got hold of a pair of scissors, he would cut his hair so that we would have to clipper it afterwards. Every single pair of scissors had to be hidden away but still he managed to sniff them out on several occasions. Once I even had to squeeze in a quick hair cut before he left for school in the morning! So for a long time Joshua sported a very short haircut. Thankfully, after several months he tired of the 'hair cutting game'. To this day we still have no idea what brought about an end to his intense dislike of hair clippers and hairdressers. If it was a sensory problem which caused him to be overly sensitive and frightened by the sound, he is certainly over it now! Who knows maybe one day he will be able to tell us. I hope so.

Of course it also goes without saying that the dentist was not one of Joshua's favourite haunts either but perhaps we can all relate to this one. The dentist certainly had his work cut out for him as far as Joshua was concerned. There would be lots of tears, screaming and a great reluctance to actually open his mouth at all, which would make his check-ups virtually impossible and highly stressful. Poor Mark would have to jam his thumb into the side of Joshua's mouth to enable the dentist to take a peek at his teeth. All the while Joshua would be biting down on Mark's thumb. OUCH! I suspect that the dentist could hear Joshua screaming in the waiting room well before he saw him. Again events took a similar turn. On one particular visit (without warning) he just seemed to be completely relaxed. Joshua did not appear to be panicky even though he knew exactly where he was going. Once in the examination room he sat down calmly. He opened his mouth when asked to allowing the dentist to examine Joshua's teeth properly, for the very first time. Joshua shocked us all by being more than accommodating with the dentist's requests. All in all though, it had taken several visits before the dentist actually got to check Joshua's teeth properly. Thankfully they were healthy. Again we were just overcome with pride at the accomplishments of our son. No, he hadn't come first in a race, or excelled in an exam or anything like that; instead he had learnt to cope with what was for him another challenging life skill. There could have been no greater reward for us that day.

You might be thinking that life for Joshua was just trekking from one life skill lesson to another; not so. There were of course lots of fun activities such as the music group which I mentioned earlier. It was a great little group that encouraged fun and learning through music and song. The kids did not only learn about music, but in a light-hearted way, they were also being trained to follow instructions. Their activities involved singing action songs and playing a variety of percussion instruments. This inevitably involved sharing and turn taking. Admittedly, it was challenging at times to keep Joshua sitting on a chair and not allow him to help himself to a toy that another child may have brought along. From Joshua's perspective it was perfectly reasonable for him to help himself to that 'Bob the builder' toy simply because he could reach it. After all, it was just sitting there and it was one of his favourite characters. He would take it with absolutely no regard at all for the distraught child to whom it actually belonged. In fact, he probably would not even look at the child's face which was communicating things that Joshua just did not understand. So to those who did not know him, he might come across as an extremely naughty and selfish child who really ought to have known better at his age! How were they to know that Joshua had very little understanding of social skills? For him it was an unfathomable area; a sea of confusion! Yes, there were weeks when I would come out of the session asking myself exactly why I was putting myself though it. The answer was always the same: I had other children and I just didn't think it fair that they all missed out. Also, Joshua enjoyed the music sessions. Even though he found the social rules difficult he still needed to comprehend something of them. Maybe this was what the experts referred to as 'mind blindness'? He wasn't necessarily being naughty by taking someone else's toy. It was not premeditated. He simply saw it and wanted it. In his mind there was just the toy and him. The child, to whom the toy actually belonged, didn't exist to him or was at best just in the background as the 'toy provider'.

So persevere we did and gradually over a period of time Joshua learnt to stay seated. Eventually Joshua could even go and choose an instrument, at the appropriate time, by himself and then swap it for another when asked to. He started to do more of the actions to the songs and would sometimes even sing at home. (Of course we didn't know it at the time but, the lady running the group also did music sessions at both the nursery and the school Joshua would eventually attend. It was a fantastic surprise and, for me, further confirmation that both the nursery and school we had chosen was the right place for him.)

I have realised that although life is hectic and the pace is forever getting faster it isn't so with Joshua. We are unable to force him to develop at a rate that is beyond him. For him change comes about when it does. The time frame is not a definite structured thing but it is flexible and adaptable. He is constantly challenging me as to what is really important in life and forcing me to question my priorities. I have come to accept that my plans are constantly being disrupted and that things very rarely run according to my agenda. In my mind my daily schedule is written in pencil, rubber at hand if needed. I try to accept each day as it comes never knowing what jewels each day will bring. Each achievement that Joshua makes I see as another precious gem to be added to the collection. In fact, in my mind, each of my children has their own collection of 'precious gems'. Some are memories, others achievements or developmental milestones and so on. They are different for each one of them and go part of the way to making them who they are. Joshua's achievements are unique to him and just as dear to me.

Joshua how is life played out through your eyes
All of the sights, the smells and the sounds?
How do they stimulate your senses?
Do they make you smile or drag you down?

Do you look forward to tomorrow
Or do you dread more of the same?
How do you cope with the hustle and bustle?
Is daily living a constant strain?

Do you tire from trying to communicate
To a world that doesn't understand?
Does it help to withdraw to somewhere within
A safe place within this alien land?

Do you long to be understood and accepted
Just the way that you are?
Is it lonely at times my precious one?
Does the journey seem just too far?

6 TIME TO ROAM!

The behaviour displayed by autistic individuals can often be misunderstood. Quite often, their coping strategies can be misinterpreted as bad behaviour or rudeness, especially when witnessed by someone who has never come across autism before. There are times when onlookers can be judgemental. Thankfully it is not something that we have experienced that often as far as Joshua is concerned. However, many people with a special needs child, autistic or otherwise, may well have encountered negative reactions somewhere along the line. For me there is one time in particular that stands out. It was when Joshua had escaped from the garden yet again. As soon as we managed to stop him from escaping one way he would simply escape by some other route. A door only had to be unlocked for seconds and if for some reason he wanted to go he would wander off, without as much as a glance behind him. On this particular occasion he had managed to get out of the front door. He had wandered up the road and was heading to who knows where. Minutes later we realised that he was not in the garden where we had thought he was and we automatically got into our 'search for Joshua mode'. Just as we were about to go off in various directions there was a knock at the door. A man was standing there with Joshua in tow. As it happened he had been driving past. He saw a small boy out on his own and he had brought him to the nearest door, which naturally was ours. Joshua walked in without as much as a 'hello'. That should have told him something. Before we could get the words out about Joshua being autistic, he proceeded to lecture us on good parenting and he was unnecessarily rude. I was so relieved that Joshua was safe that I wasn't listening too much to what he was saying. We simply thanked him and tried again to explain. It wasn't until after he had gone that his judgemental attitude and the sting of his words actually hit me. He obviously didn't have a clue regarding autism and as he wouldn't listen, unfortunately, he left none the wiser. Ironically that is the nature of autism, misunderstanding. In fact the two words go hand in hand. Not only do those suffering from autism misunderstand the workings and subtle goings on of this world but they are often totally misread themselves. What is more, their families are often misjudged because they are in so many ways living a different kind of life.

Actually we have lost count of the number of times Joshua has escaped. He would normally head towards a specific place. It might be the park, the shop or somewhere else familiar. The biggest shock came when he wandered into the local pub and boldly sat down at the bar. Amazingly enough someone recognised him and brought him home. The strange thing is that we don't really go to the local pub and we were wondering why he would have chosen to go there. Then again, when we thought about it, there were a couple of occasions one summer when we had all gone there for a meal as a family. I can only assume that Joshua was peckish! He has escaped to the pub twice and as a precaution the landlady took our number!

Whenever we think we have covered all of the available exits he simply ups his game and he comes up with a new escape route. He really is our own little 'Houdini'! As well as bedroom locks, there are also locks on the kitchen, the dining room and the windows. So to go from one room to another in our house can take time! The front door is usually locked as is the back door unless the children are playing in the garden. Despite our efforts there are still occasions when Joshua decides it's time to wander. He has been quite inventive over the years. Joshua seems to look for just the right moment when he knows everyone is occupied and then he will make his move. Even though he tends to go barefoot in the garden he prefers to wear shoes to go further a-field. So if we ever see Joshua putting his shoes on it generally means he is planning a little trip. I had thought I was a few steps ahead of him by hiding his shoes but it turns out he really isn't that fussy. He was once found cycling down the road on his sisters pink bike wearing her pink Wellington boots! On one of his little jaunts he even wore a pair of my shoes! There have been instances when Joshua has managed to outwit us even when we thought that all the windows and doors were locked. We couldn't understand how he was escaping. We then discovered that he had found out where the keys for the windows were hidden and that he was unlocking one of them when no one was looking. He would then put the keys back where he had found them and simply escape at leisure.

This is one of the bizarre things about autism. Joshua had taught himself how to open a door or window with a key. Until we actually saw him using them we simply didn't know that he knew how to. What is more, although Mark has about ten keys on his key ring Joshua knows exactly which ones to use for the front and back doors. He can find the right key quicker than any of us. There have been instances when we have all been in the garden and he has still managed to outsmart us. All it would take was for the telephone to ring or for someone to turn up at the front door. While we were preoccupied for a moment he would have pushed a bike, or anything else that would do the trick, up against the fence and he would disappear over it. If he wants to wander then his determination really is second to none! Without a doubt, Joshua's most notorious escape has to be the occasion when he managed to escape stark naked! We had just bought a free standing swimming pool for the garden and he had been taking a dip. One minute he was in the pool wearing trunks and the next he was nowhere to be seen. His trunks had been discarded on the ground. We knew that he couldn't be far away because he had been in the garden just moments before. Mark found him heading up the road without a stitch on, much to the bewilderment of the passing cars. We got him inside quickly. Ten minutes later there was a policeman knocking at the door. He had received reports that there was a naked boy heading up the road! We explained that it was our son and that he was autistic. The policeman then quickly got on his radio to call off the helicopter and the police dogs. They had been about to send a search party out for him! By coincidence, it turned out that the policeman himself had an autistic son and so was well aware of the tendency of some autistic individuals to wander off.

Of course when we look back, it is with a certain element of humour. However, our laugher only masks our awareness of the potential danger that he has unwittingly put himself in. We pray constantly that God would keep his hedge of protection around Joshua. It is our belief that it is only by the grace of God that Joshua has been found by honest people. We are under no illusions and realise that this is a very grave situation. Somehow Joshua needs to learn how dangerous it is to wander and that it really is not wise at all to go off with a total stranger. He has some idea of danger and as time has passed his understanding has grown in this area, but he still has a long way to go. I have had to try hard not to dwell on the worst case scenarios and just trust God to keep him, knowing that ultimately God can be with him always and I cannot. Thankfully, as Joshua has got older (and hopefully a bit wiser) he doesn't tend to go off on his own. In fact he has not escaped for quite some time. Long may it last!

It is hardly surprising that we have built up a collection of locks within our home. Our accumulation of locks has been gradual. We started off with a lock on the kitchen door. This was great because it meant that Joshua could no longer access the food cupboards and the fridge. So if I went upstairs, for instance, on my return I would not find Joshua pouring milk onto the carpet just for the fun of it. It was necessary and it brought much peace into our home for a while. However children grow and Joshua was no exception. In time he realised that he was tall enough to drag a chair over to the kitchen door and reach the bolt, which he did of course on a regular basis. We obviously needed something different and so we then got a lock that required a key. This was ok to start with but you had to be strict about hanging the key up or you would be forever looking for it. We were finding that it was becoming more difficult to leave things out because absolutely nothing was sacred to Joshua. He enjoyed squirting toothpaste, liquid soap, shampoo and the like all over the bathroom. If he came across a pen or paint he would not think twice about decorating a wall with some delightful smiley faces or 'finishing' one of the other children's homework. There were many tears over precious pictures, paintings, models, as well as toys which were destroyed in some way. No amount of reasoning with Joshua, or telling him off, seemed to make the slightest bit of difference. It is hard to watch and is harder still to live through. As a parent you are torn between shielding your special needs child from any resentment and your other children who are hurting, because of the seemingly senseless wreckage of their belongings. The simple things in life suddenly require a lot more thought. Gone are the days when I can just bake a cake and leave it out to cool, on the side, without shutting and locking the kitchen door. Normally when your children reach a certain age they can be trusted to leave it alone when they have been told to or, at the very least, to ask if they can have a piece. In a situation involving food being left out at home, Joshua has erased NO from his memory. He might comply for the two seconds or so after you have told him but he considers it perfectly acceptable to try again, a few seconds later. In our house baking and icing a cake before Joshua has sampled it is still quite an achievement!

One of the positive aspects of his total lack of

regard for personal possessions (if indeed there is one) is that after a while material things become less important. Now whenever we buy something new I remind myself that it could well get wrecked by Joshua. It is only a 'thing' and at the end of the day we cannot take it with us. Even so I can't expect my kids to always be that philosophical. It is still hard because after all there are some things that are precious to us that are simply irreplaceable. Those are the things that I have come to deem as more important now. You know, a picture or a model that one of your children has made or photographs for example. To find them wrecked senselessly is hard for them to take, let alone understand. To help them to cope without bitterness and resentment is a challenge. So the best thing for our family has been to find coping strategies, hence the locks on the doors. It is irritating to have to negotiate so many locks but the security far out-weights the annoyance and disappointment! The code locks on the bedrooms always require an explanation when we have people visiting for the first time!

So what about our other children? Well they have had to cope with a lot. They often get tired and frazzled parents at the end of a long day. Of course we try to minimize the negative effects that having an autistic child has on them, but with the best will in the world we are unable to shelter them completely. They are all very good with Joshua and as time passes he is interacting with them more. This just goes to show how gracious they have been with him. Joshua's autism is something that I believe has developed positive character traits in each of them. They are learning first hand that true love is unconditional and their generosity continues to amaze us. His limited language and lack of understanding are very real obstacles and at times he can still be destructive. Every year, I wonder if we will ever be able to keep flowers in the garden long enough to enjoy their beauty before Joshua starts to prune early? In spite of Joshua's relatively easy going nature there are instances when his siblings have to cope with his frustration. It is at these times that he tends to bang his head with something or, at worst, hit out at someone else. He is unable to communicate what is causing him to lash out and we are not always able to work it out ourselves. After Joshua had hit Megan one day, I later put pen to paper to try and describe this mixture of emotions that I was feeling. This is what I wrote:

'She stood before me in tears wondering exactly what she had done to provoke her brother this time. She was holding her head where the toy had hit her or should I say been thrown at her. I tried to comfort her. I too was at a loss as to what explanation to give because I knew that there was none. Not one that made sense to us anyway. I felt grief for both of my children, but for different reasons of course. I wanted to rub the pain away from my little girls head. Not just the physical pain but the emotional bruising. I also wanted to try and bridge the gap between Joshua who sometimes finds it impossible to connect with this world and the people in it. I wanted to unravel the frustration from within him because I could only assume that it was frustration that had triggered his outburst. I didn't know for sure because he could not tell me. My heart was breaking for both of them and for the inability of both parties to speak the others' language. As a mother, my instincts will me to bridge that gap but try as I might I cannot. Instead, I constantly

attempt to outwit my son and in a sense minimise the confusion for the rest of my family. The fact is that I love all of my children equally. As natural as it is for them to argue from time to time, it always hurts so much more when the strife is between Joshua and one of his siblings. At such times he is like an overgrown toddler who doesn't fully comprehend what he has done wrong. Yet still I made him face his sister and apologise. Once again I tried to make him understand that we don't hit out at people. My hope is that, over time, greater realisation will come. If anger is ever directed towards him, he sobs tears of deep pain. It is as though he doesn't understand what he has done to provoke such a response. I wonder about Joshua's future. I know that I am unable to adequately prepare him for life, or protect him from harm, the way that a mother would want to.'

The incident which inspired those thoughts was in direct contrast to the scene in our hallway, the following day. Joshua was playing beautifully with his sister. It was one of those moments I wished I had recorded but all I could do was to stare in wonder. They were each sitting on a bouncy toy. Joshua was being encouraged by his sister to bounce down the hallway with her, which he was of course eager to do. There was much enjoyment and lots of giggling. Priceless.

7 OVERLOAD!

Joshua has always loved being outside. It was for his fourth birthday that we decided to buy him a big trampoline for the garden, instead of throwing him a party. We knew that he would get so much more out of it than he would a party. He had almost worn a hole through the small one that he had indoors! Of all of the presents that we have bought for Joshua, the trampoline has probably been the biggest hit. He gets so much pleasure out of it and it is lovely to see him having so much fun. The added bonus being that it is something he can enjoy with siblings and friends. It has also aided his social development. He is happy to play on the trampoline on his own but he much prefers it when there are other children bouncing with him. Joshua's eye contact is amazing when he is bouncing and he seems to be able to connect more easily with others who are sharing one of his favourite activities. His sense of balance is incredible and he is a real natural. So that year Joshua's birthday was more of an intimate affair. It was celebrated by close family with lots of ice cream, cake, candles, presents and the like. As it was the summer holidays the children were able to spend a lot of time outdoors. So whenever Joshua had the opportunity he would be out on the trampoline. I remember that summer as being a very peaceful time in our lives. As a family we were becoming more accustomed to life with an autistic child. We seemed to have entered a period of greater calm; or maybe it was just the 'calm before the storm'. It was some time after Joshua's birthday that I noticed a few red spots on Joshua's face. They didn't look like anything serious and almost resembled chicken pox because they seemed to have a bit of fluid in the centre. I really wasn't that concerned. If it was chicken pox it would have been good to get it over and done with while he was young. If it wasn't then I assumed the spots would disappear as quickly as they had come. However, after a few days not only were they still there but the patch of spots had got slightly bigger. The spots had not spread to any other part of his body. They were still just on his face. They didn't appear to be itchy or to be causing Joshua any discomfort but they did not seem to be clearing up. That summer we took the children to Legoland for the first time; it was a great day. On the way back I noticed that the red patch on Joshua's face seemed slightly worse. Call it a mother's intuition if you like but I had an uneasy feeling about it. So we stopped off at the local health centre to get a nurse to have a look at it. The nurse who saw Joshua's face seemed to think it was some kind of insect bite but she said that Joshua should definitely be seen by the doctor. So we took her advice and booked a doctor's appointment. The doctor wasn't too sure what it was exactly. He didn't think it was too much to worry about and gave me some cream to apply to the area. Days later, it was obvious that the cream was having no effect at all because the rash still wasn't healing. If anything it was still getting worse. Another ointment was prescribed and eventually, after several weeks, the spots cleared up leaving a red patch where they had been. The patch of skin was no longer smooth but looked like scar tissue. It was only when the redness had faded that you could see clearly that the affected area of Joshua's skin had completely lost its pigmentation. So he now had a white patch of skin surrounded by his natural tan. The contrast in skin colour was further exaggerated by the fact that he had developed a sun tan, over the summer months. Mark and I assumed that eventually his skin would return to normal. Instead, further white patches started to appear. He seemed to be losing pigmentation on his face in small areas. Joshua already had so many problems but the one thing that Joshua had always had was his gorgeous good looks, but now even the skin on his face was marred. Looking at Joshua's patchy skin I felt doubly cheated. It just didn't seem fair. A referral to a dermatologist followed because the doctors suspected it could be 'Vitiligo', a skin condition where patches of skin simply lose their natural pigmentation.

More appointments and more waiting followed. The specialists were still not sure what the problem was as, in their opinion, Vitiligo didn't normally behave in this way. They were mystified as to the role that the rash had played. We were advised to be doubly careful when Joshua was out in the sun. He had to be smothered in the highest factor sun cream and wear a hat at all times. He would go off with his sun cream on in the morning and have it liberally applied, several times during the day, because his skin had become so sensitive. It put extra pressure on us to always remember to bring a hat and to ensure that he wore it. Needless to say he wasn't keen. If he was at school and the sun came out I would wonder whether he was outside and, if so, did he have his sun cream and hat on? Joshua's skin seemed to be so sensitive that it didn't even have to be that warm for his skin to be affected. As the weather got cooler it brought some relief because it meant that Joshua's skin wasn't so much at risk. His tan faded over the winter months and slowly his skin seemed to be returning to normal. The contrast in skin colour wasn't so obvious. By the beginning of the following spring Mark and I took Joshua to see the specialist. His skin had virtually returned to normal. It looked as though all the hard work had paid off. Sadly life is not always as straightforward as we would like it to be. Literally just weeks after Joshua had been signed off by the dermatologist we were all enjoying a day out. We had taken the children to a couple of museums and then out for lunch. Although it was only the end of March it was one of those freakishly sunny days that reminded you of the summer months to come. I remember us walking through some beautiful gardens and enjoying some unhurried time. I smiled down at Joshua whose hand I was holding. The smile on my face soon faded. Was it just my imagination? He seemed to have lost the pigment in his lower eyelashes and most of his eyebrow, on the right side of his face? I examined his face again and immediately went cold. I could see that there were several bright white skin patches. This time, not only did he have all of the old patches back again but a few new ones had also appeared. At that point I could have sobbed right there in the city centre. Maybe I was over-reacting but we had worked so hard to combat the skin damage. It all appeared to have been in vain and it seemed to be much worse than it had been before. On closer inspection we noticed that a white hair lock had started to develop, in addition to the de-pigmented area of the eyebrow and eyelashes. I was absolutely beside myself. A few weeks ago he had been given the all clear and now this. We were not certain exactly when the skin and hair had started to lose their colour but we hadn't noticed it until that day. Admittedly we had been in and out of the sunshine for a while. Was his skin really that sensitive to the sun?

The tranquillity that I had felt earlier seemed to drain away as I made a frantic phone call to the dermatology department. They were very understanding and the receptionist sorted out an appointment for Joshua to be seen again. So a few weeks later we were back with the dermatologist who was really surprised to see how his condition had deteriorated. She took photos of the affected areas. We were also given a cream, a fairly new medication, which had been shown to have quite good results at re-pigmenting the skin. The dermatologist did however explain that because it was a fairly new product they were not sure what the long term effects were. There was even a possibility that with prolonged use it could be carcinogenic. The trouble was that where his skin had lost its pigment it was more vulnerable anyway.

I was devastated on Joshua's behalf but grateful that he was unaware of what was happening. So the battle began again to stop the sun's rays from harming Joshua's skin, while still allowing this outdoors loving child to enjoy and explore the world outside. It is amazing how adaptable children are. He soon came to accept that he had to keep his hat on all the time when outside, sun or no sun. On the occasions when he discarded it he was told to go and put his hat on and he would comply. He also got used to having cream applied more regularly than any of the other children. On top of this he had to have his special ointment applied first thing in the morning, on the patches, before his sun cream and before he went to bed at night. The dermatologist was still puzzled by Joshua's skin and thought it would be good if Joshua was seen by a panel of skin experts. She asked us if we would agree to come to the hospital, where a team of dermatologists would take turns observing Joshua's skin and getting some background information on his condition. Of course we said yes because we wanted as much information as possible. So weeks later, Mark and I were sitting in a hospital room with Joshua and answering endless questions. We were there for quite a while and Joshua coped extremely well as doctors came in and peered at his face curiously while trying hard to communicate with him. No major revelations resulted from all of this. It looked as though it had to be some type of segmented Vitiligo, since there didn't appear to be any other obvious explanation. Joshua's dermatologist was extremely thorough and left no stone unturned. She also referred Joshua to the genetics department. They carried out tests to find out if his skin problems were linked to certain hereditary conditions, normally associated with a white hair lock. We needed to be sure for the wellbeing of all of our children. After much testing (including an MRI scan) thankfully this was ruled out.

There are times when life seems to be just one big hospital appointment. More of your life seems to be spent in hospital waiting rooms than anywhere else. It is hard for any child to be constantly waiting around in a hospital or doctor's surgery. It is doubly hard when that child has no understanding as to why he is even there. It was tough on Joshua when he had to have his MRI scan. He was unable to eat or drink anything for a long period of time, because the only way they were going to keep him still was to give him a general anaesthetic. I won't forget the moment that he went under. It was like watching all the life drain out of him as he went completely limp and lifeless. As it turned out all of the prodding and poking was in vain, but at least it ruled out the possibility of anything else.

So what was Joshua's skin like at its worst? Well, he had a big white patch on his forehead which continued down the right side of his nose. There was literally a line running down his nose, white on one side but tanned on the other. The worst area was around his right eye. It was his right eyebrow and eyelashes that had partially lost their colour. He looked as though he had a big white patch round his eye which was outlined by a dark brown jagged line (much darker than his normal skin colour). The white area continued underneath the eye and spread to the outer corner of his eye all the way to his hair line where it joined forces with a white hair lock. In time, the harsh jagged brown areas, that seemed to have too much pigment, gradually began to fade. The white sections, being treated with the cream from the dermatologist, started to re-pigment very slowly in parts. It seemed to take an eternity but bit by bit small patches of his skin were returning to normal and the white sections seemed to be shrinking in size.

At present Joshua's skin is still patchy but not nearly as noticeable. We still need to apply sun cream liberally and he still needs to wear a hat. His condition is always worse in the summer and but not so noticeable in the winter. However each year his skin seems to get a fraction better. In the early days I would feel myself starting to panic if Joshua was out in the sun and I wasn't with him. I have had to adopt a more relaxed attitude for my own sanity, because there really is nothing I can do about the sun shining! There will always be times when we are caught out because that is life. Quite recently we went on holiday to France and the weather was great. It was the first time that we had taken our children abroad. We thought it would make sense to choose somewhere with similar weather to our own because of Joshua's skin. One of the highlights of the holiday was the outdoor pool. Obviously this was an occasion where Joshua quite clearly could not wear a hat and his skin, although well protected by cream, did start to look very patchy again. The dark jagged lines on his skin started to reappear. We also noticed that once again there was a line down the centre of his nose. This was something that we hadn't seen for a long time and it did feel as though we were back tracking.

On a positive note though Joshua and his brothers and sister were having the best of times and I am sure they will always remember that holiday. Joshua was taking everything in his stride and he wasn't fazed at all by the unfamiliar language or eating out in new restaurants. We had travelled over by car on the Eurotunnel and the car journey, once in France, had been a long one. Yet still he didn't fuss because he knew that we were going on holiday. So there was plenty to smile about and I knew that I had a choice to make. Either I spent the entire holiday uptight and worried about his skin or I just did the very best that I could and then let it go. I chose to do the latter and in doing so felt that this was just another small step in my trusting God with Joshua. I could never have been as relaxed about it a year before. God was able to give me peace in the midst of the situation and he had brought me to a place where I was able to accept it. Thankfully we found that during the weeks following our holiday the patchiness became less obvious again.

8 DARING TO LOOK FORWARD

There is nothing at all special about Mark and myself. It is our faith that keeps us from caving in emotionally. That is what enables us to keep putting one foot in front of the other, when everything within us is screaming at us to stop. God is the one who keeps us together as a family when things are just too much. Where else do you find the energy to keep going when you are building your own house, have three children going to school sixteen miles from home, while another goes to school 8 miles in the opposite direction? This is while trying to run a business and of course be there for your children. Most of the time you just get on with it but occasionally you stop and wonder how much longer you can walk this road, before you end up in a state of collapse. I am not at all surprised that so many marriages break up under the strain of it all. Having a special needs child puts enormous pressure on your marriage; let us not even begin talking about the tiredness. Having children is tiring in itself but having an autistic child can sometimes take you to levels of tiredness and busyness that you didn't even think were possible. There are many people who walk part of the journey with you. Our children are blessed with grandparents who have chosen to do just that. They do not sit on the side-lines and observe but they are very much involved in our lives. My mother helps to look after Joshua and the other children, when she is able to. Granddad will collect Joshua from school when we cannot, for which we are so appreciative. Of course they do so much more than that. They constantly give of themselves, but perhaps one of the most precious things that they do for us all is to pray. I know that we are constantly in their prayers.

I often wonder how people cope when their children barely sleep or are even more demanding and more difficult than Joshua. I know that there are so many people out there who are coping with extremely challenging behaviours that most of us couldn't even begin to imagine. I listen, with absolute amazement, when others share their stories because I am truly in awe of their capacity to love and to give, even in the most desperate of circumstances. The conclusion I come to, again and again, is that they must be very special people to be able to give so generously, although I am sure they do not see themselves that way. They probably have never even stopped to consider it.

I can honestly say that we are all being deeply challenged and changed by the whole experience. If I see a child misbehaving and a parent struggling to take control I don't assume it is bad parenting or that the child is being particularly naughty. These days I would be more inclined to send up a quick prayer for them. We cannot always see what is wrong with a person simply from the outward appearance. They may be battling against something that we are totally unaware of, so I try not to judge because I know what it is like to have a child who is often misunderstood. There are days when Joshua seems to be much more a part of us and this world; hope seems to rise up within my heart. This is inevitably followed by a period when he seems more remote than ever and despair seems to extinguish some of my optimism. Is

it possible to describe with mere words the true depth
of all that emotion.….?

Joshua sometimes you see me
Sometimes you don't
Some days you hear me
Other days you won't

You are my child and I love you so
Such depths of love you may never know
Be assured that for you I am always there
Your name my love is my daily prayer

Those days that I fail you please forgive
As I try to arm you with the tools to live
When it looks as though my grace is running dry
When deep despair seems to engulf my sky

When all around me seems so black
When hopelessness seems to be breaking my back
A ray of hope comes seeping through
Hope from above, from my God for you

He picks me up and dusts me down
He comforts me without a sound
His peace pierces my very core
Without him my hope would be no more

I think of the struggle so many are going through
day after day. It is often a struggle that they are unable
to win and one that is slowly wearing them down.
Who can help them? I have an amazing vision of a
special needs school, or centre, which would not only
provide stimulation for the child (in the area of

socialisation and learning) but would feed them spiritually too. It wouldn't just be concerned with the child but in fact the wellbeing of the whole family. Having special needs within a family can bring with it enormous demands and any support is invaluable. How amazing it would be to have people who could support you in prayer for your child and family. I would love to see the peace of God penetrate the lives of these children and their families because I think it is so very much needed.

For my husband it has been a different journey in some ways. As I have already mentioned he has a Downs syndrome brother who is two years younger than himself. His brother has all sorts of learning difficulties. Therefore his perspective on Joshua is different to mine. He knows what it is like to have a sibling who is different and has experienced first-hand the destruction of his belongings. He remembers what it is like to want to play with someone who simply doesn't know how to. For him it was almost like being an only child. His brother had numerous medical problems as well and Mark spent much of his younger years in hospital waiting rooms. In addition to this he himself had problems at school, partly due to dyslexia which was not diagnosed until he was fifteen. One of his biggest regrets is that he did not receive the help he so badly needed at school. For him school was not a safe place.

It was not until my first pregnancy that I began to realise, more clearly, how having a special needs brother had affected Mark. Up until then he had never really talked about it at length. However it emerged that one of his greatest fears for us as a couple was that we too could have a Down's child.

Surely there was no way that God would allow anything like that to happen? Little did I know what was in store for us? I am sure that there have been times when Mark has looked at Joshua but has really seen his brother. For him our experience of autism as a family brings back a whole host of memories. Of course they are memories of a different time. They have nothing to do with Joshua and I know that. Although Mark also knows this, inevitably memories from his earlier experiences sometimes trickle into the present. As Mark himself says, 'I have so many mixed emotions. I love and care for Joshua dearly. He is my son; yet I constantly battle with the fact that he is special needs and that I feel robbed. My heart goes out to my other children because I know how it feels from their perspective. There is nothing I can do to change the situation and I feel so helpless. I would do anything to prevent my children from experiencing what I went through as a child but, on the other hand, there isn't a mountain I wouldn't climb to help Joshua.' As a couple we have to try to keep moving forward. All we can do is what we think is best and continue asking God to show us which way to go. There are days when it is like walking through patchy fog and we have no idea which direction we are heading in. We feel despondent and it is as though we are on a treadmill going absolutely nowhere. Then there are those moments of pure joy when you can see the fruits of your efforts and the graciousness of God.

It is all too easy to feel weighed down by the problems associated with having Joshua and I suppose it is bound to happen from time to time. However, as with all sorts of trying and stretching situations, there are always positives which spring up unexpectedly. Having Joshua has definitely changed the dynamics of our family. We would not be who we are today if we were without him. God, for reasons unknown to us, has allowed us to experience our own world of autism. I often look back at photos taken before Joshua was born. My ideals and priorities were very different. I was much more bothered about what other people thought back then. Now if my main focus was how other people saw us as a family I wouldn't bother getting out of bed in the morning. To survive this marathon called 'our life' we have become much more laid back, because quite frankly our sanity requires it! If I worried about every item that was destroyed or every time something got spilt I would be a total wreck. It has been and still is a daily challenge and I am sure that on many occasions I am in fact a total wreck! More often than not I can now see the signs. I have had to learn to send out an arrow prayer quickly and wait for God to do for me what I cannot do for myself. All I know is that it is harder to cope when I am completely wound up, than when I am relaxed. My coping strategy might be to shut myself away in the kitchen, have a cup of tea and a few moments to myself. The more simple things in life like peace and joy are too precious to take for granted and we are learning that they are not necessarily the fruits of a stress-free life.

As for Mark and I we always try to set aside some time. We might go for a coffee or have lunch. Whatever we do, it is simply nice to spend time together. It is hard enough for us and I am simply in awe of those who are coping alone. There is such a need to get alongside people who are parenting on their own, so that they are not just left to get on with it. They need time out and support too! It is uplifting to meet and talk to others who are going through a similar experience. I think that when you have a special needs child you are much more aware of those who are also being challenged in similar ways. Let's face it though all children are special and they can all be demanding! They don't have to be 'special needs' to be hard work. Parenting is a tall order and not for the faint hearted! Yet, I have also found it to be the most rewarding, amazing and meaningful experience ever. One of the challenges with autism, that I have found, is that most of the tried and tested ways that work for my other children do not necessarily work with Joshua. Sometimes they do but it is normally a case of trial and error. The autistic spectrum is so wide that it would be highly unlikely to find another autistic child just like my son. It is good to hear how other people have tackled certain issues because it gives you ideas.

On one of our trips to Centre Parcs we were looking on as our eldest son went tree trekking. Standing near us was another family with children and they too were watching proudly as their son took part. Mark and I were keeping an eye on Joshua who was getting restless. He was bored and totally oblivious to the fact that his brother was several feet above him, so we took turns to entertain him. Later I bumped into the same family and was able to chat briefly with the mother. She had realised straight away that Joshua was autistic because her son (who had been tree-trekking) was also autistic. She then shocked me by saying that he had been just like Joshua when younger. She recalled how much hard work it had been but said it was worth it and encouraged me to hang on in there. Those few words meant the world to me. I looked at her and told her that their hard work had obviously paid off because their son was an absolute credit to them. That short conversation encouraged me to keep going. Isn't encouragement such a precious and vital gift?

Life is forever changing and as we look to the future we know that there are more crossroads ahead. Although Joshua is doing well in school we realise that the time will come when he will need to move on. They do an absolutely fantastic job and he has had supportive teachers in every class. As for his TA's, they really have gone above and beyond the call of duty. As a result we have never had any concerns when Joshua has been in their care. They have had such a great relationship with him and a real heart for him. Although it is true that Joshua is maturing and learning all the time, the fact is that the academic and social gap between him and his peers is widening. While they are learning quickly how to be mature and more responsible young people, Joshua still has to be reminded to be quiet at the appropriate times, or not to throw something on the floor when frustrated. He still doesn't get this complicated thing called 'life' and all those unspoken rules that he is supposed to have learned by now. It is easier to teach a child when to sit or stand, at the appropriate time, but much harder to teach them that it is not acceptable to take your trousers off during P.E., because you sat on a wet patch. It is easy to physically stop a child from running off but harder to make them understand the reasons why they shouldn't wander off, when they simply do not have the level of understanding required. In many ways Joshua is interacting with his siblings better than ever. He is beginning to understand different emotions and why we have them at different times, but progress is still slow. Teaching Joshua abstract concepts is a huge challenge. We don't want him to be attending a mainstream school but to be so limited by his autism that he spends much of his time on his own anyway. What would be the point in that? So over the next year we need to make a decision regarding his education. He has gained so much from being around 'normal functioning' children. In addition to this he has had one to one help the entire time he has been there. Sadly, if he goes to a special school he would lose his one to one help, but would benefit from the opportunities and activities that would probably only be available in a special needs setting.

I often look back over the journey so far and I can see that Joshua's life has been enriched by so many different experiences. For instance, he has been on all of the school trips and has not been fazed by the fact that he was dressed for school but not going to school. We were able to accompany him, as helpers, on all but one of his school outings. For the most recent one neither Mark nor I were free and it was suggested that he went on the school coach, with his TA's. I must admit I wasn't too sure initially because normally the three of us would meet them there, having travelled up in our car. In the end, we all decided it would be a good experience for him. He definitely rose to the challenge and coped admirably. All of these events have added to his time at school, in a positive way. He is included in most things.

Life certainly is not humdrum in our family and

most of the time you never know what Joshua is going to get up to next. For instance, while on holiday we were having a drink in a cafe. The other children were drinking iced fruit juices with umbrellas and straws. Joshua had chosen to drink water but seemed to be taking a real interest in these colourful concoctions and it was obvious that he wanted to taste one. He sipped it but then disaster struck and it fell crashing to the floor. We were so encouraged that he had tried something new and since it was an accident we replaced it. He seemed really excited when this second drink arrived and again took a sip. We all settled back in our chairs and continued to relax. However, seconds later the drink, followed by the cup was flying through the air towards the bin. Joshua could hardly contain his excitement when this drink too crashed to the floor, going absolutely everywhere. So tell me what do you do? Well after the initial shock all we could do was laugh. Luckily it didn't hit anyone and no one seemed to notice because we were outside, right in the corner. Joshua had confused us again. He had so enjoyed the experience of the first drink spilling everywhere that he was desperate to re-enact the scene. That would never have occurred to us but isn't that one of the mysteries of autism, 'confusion'.

As far as food and drinks are concerned we have been extremely blessed with Joshua, who has a good diet and eats a fairly wide range of healthy food. As he has got older his range of food has increased and he is forever surprising us by trying new things. One of his dislikes however has always been fizzy drinks which certainly isn't a bad thing. So if he went to a party and they were serving fizzy drinks he would have water or still juice. It confused him if the water was served in a coke cup. He would simply refuse to drink it. He still thought it contained fizzy drink even if he could see the contents of the cup! After a long while we were able to persuade him to at least try it. He realised then that the writing on the cup didn't always correspond to what was in it. A valuable lesson I think!

We often remind ourselves just how far Joshua has come, even if at times progress has been painstakingly slow. It seems a long time since Joshua's first day at nursery. Back then he was scared and probably bewildered. His virtually non-existent communication skills presented a huge challenge. I remember saying to God back then how much easier it would be if only Joshua could verbalise his basic needs. For us to have a child who could actually say 'water' when they wanted 'water' would put an end to so much of the frustration, that his lack of speech brought. 'If he could just ask for what he wanted, well, that would be a start,' I remember praying. It suddenly occurred to me that a year or so after I had prayed that prayer Joshua had started doing just that. It had been a bit of an 'off the cuff' prayer really and the answer had gone almost unnoticed by me, because the progress had been so gradual. In fact Joshua had gone beyond what I had prayed for and was starting to verbalise his emotions. For instance he would tell us that he was sad if he had hurt himself. Of course progress in this area is still slow and there are much younger children who are able to communicate their feelings far better than Joshua can. Nevertheless, if I have learnt anything it is to be grateful for the small steps and to avoid comparing him to other children, because he will never be them. He will always be Joshua. We are learning to rejoice in his personal milestones and to always expect more. We try to make the most of the positive experiences. For instance eating out as a family is a much more relaxed affair. Joshua is generally well behaved because eating out is something that he enjoys. He has a better understanding of what is expected of him now and will often ask if we can 'go and get something to eat'. Having said that, we know we cannot afford to become complacent because it is when we do that Joshua tends to seize the opportunity!

It was the end of yet another school day. The sun was shining brightly. As I was driving I could not help but be amazed at God's creation. I took in the beauty of the countryside as I sped past. It was as though I was just soaking in the presence of God. I was on my way to pick Joshua up from school. I arrived and got out of the car to join the mass of parents, also on their way to pick up their children. I spotted Joshua who had already come out and was standing with his helper. She explained that he had had a great afternoon but an unsettled morning. Apparently he had been very tearful and had been throwing things. To crown it all he had thrown his arms in the air and accidentally caught a little girl on the head. She had been startled at the time and had cried. This wasn't what I had wanted to hear but such is life. Joshua was made to say sorry and I was assured that the little girl was fine. She knew he hadn't meant to hurt her. His helper was concerned that he wasn't himself and she wanted to know if I could think of anything that might have caused him to feel out of sorts. Her guess was as good as mine. At home he seemed ok and there was certainly nothing, out of the ordinary, happening that I could put my finger on. His sister was not very well and I wondered if he too was coming down with a cold. Unfortunately Joshua couldn't enlighten us. Oh he could tell me if he had a wobbly tooth or a cut on his leg but nothing more complicated than that. We wandered back to the car and as I caught sight of mothers rushing home with their children I suddenly realised how much I had changed. There would have been a time when I would have been devastated by the fact that Joshua's morning, at school, had not been great. Although it certainly did nothing to lift my spirits, I had come to accept that sometimes life with an autistic child was like that. This was a situation over which I had very little control. Oh I could help with the practicalities such as which school he attended and the day to day running of his life, but once again I was painfully aware that I couldn't get into his head. Yes he was an extremely demonstrative child. I would be hard pushed to keep count of the number of hugs that Joshua gave me, but this was love of a different kind. He couldn't explain it, even if he could go part way to showing it. There was clearly a strong bond between Joshua and his loved ones but we couldn't begin to talk about it with him. I could feel the weariness hovering over me and so on the way home I just prayed. I needed to talk to the only One who would understand exactly how I was feeling, even before the words had left my mouth. I told Him just how hopeless everything seemed at times and how little I felt I could do. I knew that I could throw myself into doing all I could for Joshua and still not do the impossible, which was to pull him out from where he

111

was. It was something that I still had to learn to accept, bit by miniscule bit.

My thoughts turned to a conversation that I had had with my other children. I had asked them to describe life with Joshua. This is what they said:

'Sometimes I think he limits what we can do.'

'I don't like it when he runs away.'

'He is annoying because when he comes into our rooms he wrecks the place.'

'Whenever mum makes a cake he takes a bite when he shouldn't.'

'It is sometimes good because we get to jump the queue in places like Legoland.'

'I like it when he plays on the trampoline with us.'

'I love it when he calls us to play with him outside on the seesaw and swings.'

'To me Joshua is normal. He is my brother and we all love him.'

Oh to see life through a child's eyes!

Many lessons have been learnt despite the fact that there are still mountains to climb. Yes even though there are times when I feel that I simply cannot carry on anymore I know I am not alone. God himself walks with us, part carrying us, along the way. No, I do not know what the future holds but He does. Whatever is around the corner for us as a family He will be in it with us. My faith allows me to always have hope in the future even when the future, humanly speaking, looks bleak. I know that Joshua has a future in God that is tailor made for him. Having Joshua has forced me to dig deeper than I ever thought was possible. I guess when you are in a crisis situation it really is sink or swim. However with God I don't have to sink because He is my life line. No matter how hard or how bad things seem He is always by my side. I weep on his shoulder often and He is my support. Yes, I have a loving family and friends but it is God who I ultimately depend on. No one can usurp his place and without Him I am no more. I have experienced God breaking into the most desperate situations in remarkable ways and when I am feeling fragile I remind myself of those times. God never promised me a perfect or easy life but he has promised never to leave me. We do not keep going because there is something special about us but simply because there is something special about our God. Perhaps I am in a place where I can see this more clearly now? Before Joshua I didn't realise how little we know as people. Yes I had studied and got some good qualifications. I had held down good jobs, but what of them if I couldn't get into Joshua's thinking. I consider myself to be a reasonably good mother but that too counted for very little with Joshua. I have come to realise how small I am and how powerless I am to change things. Every good thing that I do and achieve is only because God has enabled me to. He has given me life and I have come to realise more fully that each day, hour and moment is a gift from above. So yes, I marvel at the sunlight glinting through the trees and I stand in awe of the One who gave my Joshua life. Yet I always remind myself that He is the same God who created this world and who gives hope to the hopeless. Yes, He is indeed my God and I will continue to praise Him; with Him by my side I can face tomorrow. As for Joshua, his future is God's secret for now but we press on with hope.

Photos, memories and images in my mind
Of days already spent, gone, behind

In blissful ignorance I carelessly lived my days
Not for a moment realising everything would change

I thought that I knew you well until one day
Your ears no longer understood the words I tried to
say

It hurt that your eyes would no longer meet my own
Communication with you was like getting blood out
of a stone

You appeared to be lost somewhere inaccessible to
me
Shutters closed, door locked but where was the key?

But as I tried hard to pierce your gaze with my own
It was as though you were in a special place all alone

Where? I did not know and could not seem to find
out
Surely God alone knows your exact whereabouts

But this, I know above all other things
The warmth, the love to my heart you bring

I often wonder if you will ever know
How much we all love you so

FINALLY, FOR ALL OF THOSE 'SPECIAL'
FAMILIES OUT THERE:
May you experience encouragement to keep moving
forward; an abundance of peace so real that it is
almost tangible and love that will never run dry.

ABOUT THE AUTHOR

Hermione Woodley lives with her husband and four children. Her son Joshua was diagnosed with autism at the age of three, catapulting their family into totally unfamiliar territory. She is committed to helping Joshua reach his full potential and encouraging her family to be all that they can be.

Printed in Great Britain
by Amazon.co.uk, Ltd.,
Marston Gate.